MW01290173

Toxic Light

Cover Picture: The filtered solar radiation from sunglasses may be able to impact your health. Scratches, imperfections and smears may cause light interference.

Contents

Introduction

Toxic light is a new field of research into human health. Can light really be toxic? Yes, and it may be the driving force behind much of the illness and disease in modern society. This book could potentially save your life and drastically improve your health and mind.

We will take a look into the various forms of light and assess them for their ability to impact health. Something as simple as your household lighting may be able to affect you. Random pains or tiredness? It may be the light in your environment.

Light is one of the least understood aspects of nature and arguably the most important. We will start out by examining sunlight and then move onto the many sources of artificial lights that are present today. Light is almost everywhere and we will see that it has many different forms, even though they look the same to the human eye. We will look into the health aspects of light and how it may be affecting you.

We will investigate the amount of daily natural light that your body needs to be healthy and you may be surprised by the type of light that you need and also the number of hours of exposure that we come up with. By the end of the book you will have a good understanding of the different types of lighting and most importantly, the types of lighting to avoid.

This book contains the very latest research on light and the human environment. It should be viewed as the current ideas on a new branch of scientific study and the contents are subject to review by the scientific community.

The author and publisher accept no liability whatsoever for any of the contents and the book is published in the spirit of unrestricted access to the latest ideas and scientific theories in a changing world.

You should always consult with a licensed and certified medical professional on any aspects of health and disease.

Sun

Our closest star at just 93 million miles from Earth. A giant nuclear reactor that appears at sunrise every day, warms us and gives light to our lives until sunset. It does this every day without fail.

The Sun is so close to us that we can tap into its nuclear energy through the light and warmth that it radiates. Solar power technology has matured and we are now starting to widely use this resource for our energy needs.

The Sun sends us approximately 1,366 watts per square meter (W/m^2) of energy to the Earth and we call this "irradiance", the measure of solar radiation power. We lose some of this energy through atmospheric effects, such as scattering and absorption. By the time it gets to sea level, about 17% of the energy has disappeared if the Sun was directly overhead, also called "zenith". We now have about 1,130 watts per square meter left of the energy and this is a high amount of power.

The Sun is only directly overhead at the tropics in summer time. Any places outside of the tropics will never see the Sun at zenith. Instead it will be at a lower angle and we need to know how this affects the energy it creates at ground level. We need to introduce a concept called "air mass".

Air mass is a measurement of how thick the atmosphere is when looking at an astronomical object. In our case we are interested in the Sun.

If you increase air mass then you will reduce the power level due to the solar radiation passing through more of the atmosphere. Air mass increases as you head towards the poles and this will cause a reduction in power received from the Sun at sea level. Air mass will change with the seasons and the two extremes for air mass will be winter solstice and summer solstice when outside of the tropics.

So our average irradiance at sea level is 1,130 W/m^2 in the tropics, or is it? Actually, no it isn't. There is another factor to consider: Reflections. Reflections can cause irradiance to increase significantly. There are many types of reflections that can increase irradiance and we will look into these in later chapters. "Albedo" is the correct name for this effect.

So is this the only power increase? No, we have another: Altitude. The higher up we get into the sky from sea level, the less atmosphere that the Suns rays have to pass through to reach the ground. So we will be able to receive more than 1,130 W/m^2 on average at higher elevations when the Sun is at zenith.

So is this it? No, there is another: Atmospherics. The atmosphere can vary in its transparency. Sometimes more energy will arrive at the ground from Space and at other times it will be less. It all depends on the atmosphere and its content, such as dust.

So as you can see, solar radiation power is a complex equation of items that can affect irradiance values and these values are always changing based on the environment and weather.

When we measure irradiance over a time period, such as a day, we call this insolation. Insolation is usually quoted in watts per square meter per day. The National Renewable Energy Laboratory (NREL) has produced many graphs that show insolation values around the world. Knowing insolation values is very useful in calculating the solar radiation power levels over the year in locations around the Earth.

This book is aimed at increasing awareness of these factors so that you can make informed decisions about solar radiation power and how it interacts with human health. We will now look into the various factors that you should know about.

Sunlight

Sunlight is made up of lots of photons that were generated at the Sun in nuclear reactions. A photon has some of the properties of a wave and some of the properties of a particle. Photon's are energy and humans know this energy as sunburn (ultraviolet), light and heat (infrared).

Sunlight can have polarity. This can occur when it passes through a filter or is reflected from a surface. Most humans will know light polarization as a type of sunglasses that can be purchased. These cut down on reflections (glare) from surfaces and bodies of water by using a polarized filter coating.

Light comes in many forms. Some of these are parallel light, semi-parallel light, non-parallel light, diffracted light and interference light. Basically sunlight travels in parallel, semi-parallel light is directional light that has started to scatter and non-parallel light is scattered light that travels in all directions. Diffracted light occurs when the light passes over an object which causes spreading light waves to occur and interference light is made up of spreading light waves that have started to cross into each other and interact.

Parallel light is produced by the Sun and is generally referred to by optical engineers as collimated light. A direct view of the Suns disk in the sky is parallel light.

Sunlight is regarded as powerful and in the wrong situation it can be harmful to human health. Most people will be familiar with the medical advice to not look directly at the Sun. The Sun is very powerful when viewed directly with the human eye. If the Sun is reflected from a flat mirror or precision engineered flat surface, this reflection is still parallel due to the Suns shape still being visible.

Semi-parallel light is a directional form of light that has some scattering in it. An image cannot be seen but it has maintained its ability to be directed. It is a powerful reflection. The Sun reflecting off water would be a good description of this type of light.

Non-parallel light is scattered light that travels in random directions. This is the desirable configuration of light sources for humans. No image of the original source of light can be seen nor are there any bright patches of reflected sunlight.

If the Sun is reflected from a surface that scatters light and the Sun cannot be seen, then this is semi-parallel or non-parallel light.

Diffraction is caused by obstacles in the path of the parallel light. The Sun can be seen to bleed into the object when it is photographed.

Toxic Light © Steven Magee

The best way to describe interference light is to direct you to images of light. Interference light shows up as rings around light sources and also crosses with the light source at the center when they are photographed. This can commonly be seen when watching movies of pop concerts.

Diffraction and interference effects are what the forest canopy produces.

A diagram of how the interference effect is formed from light waves intersecting can be found on the next page. The light waves encounter an obstacle or object and this causes diffraction. Diffraction just means that the light waves have started to spread outwards from the obstacle. Interference occurs when the spreading waves start interacting with each other.

Toxic Light © Steven Magee

Interference Diagram

The light waves arrive in parallel and expand outwards when they pass through the two apertures. Interference is produced where the waves intersect. This is seen as the bright and dark bands on the right. The dark is destructive and the bright is constructive interference.

For more information on interference:
http://electron9.phys.utk.edu/optics421/modules/m5/Interference.htm

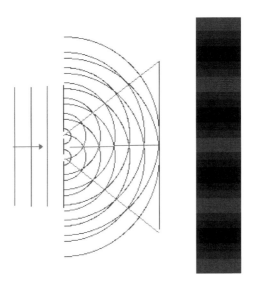

14

Solar radiation is broad spectrum radiation. This means that it contains many different types of frequencies of energy. The largest sources of energy are:

- Ultraviolet (UV)
- Optical
- Infrared (IR)

In addition to these it contains other frequencies of energy, many of which are not effectively documented by the medical profession. The effects of the content of broad spectrum solar radiation on the human body are not fully understood. Until broad spectrum solar radiation is understood, it pays to exercise caution around it.

The power levels of ground based solar radiation are not too different from that of Space. The atmosphere only absorbs about seventeen percent of the Space solar radiation energy at zenith. The frequency spectrum of the ground based solar radiation is very similar to that of Space with a just a few of the frequencies that are contained in the solar radiation spectrum being largely absorbed by the atmosphere.

The diagram on the next page shows the solar radiation spectrum power levels.

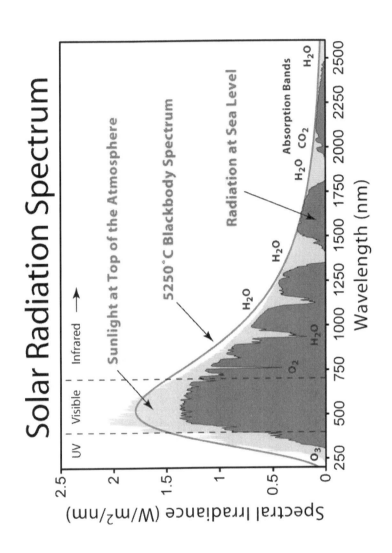

Modified Solar Radiation Spectrum

As we saw from the solar radiation spectrum graph, solar radiation is made up of many different forms of energy that make up the spectrum of solar radiation. This spectrum can be modified in a number of ways:

- Filtering
- Diffraction and interference effects
- Reflections

Filtering is what happens when solar radiation passes through something like the atmosphere, water or glass. Filtering will remove certain elements of the solar radiation spectrum and may reduce the power levels of those that pass through the filter. The result is a different spectrum of solar radiation of a lower overall power level.

Diffraction and interference effects may remove some parts of the spectrum and replace them with newly created spectrum elements from the interference effects. Interference may also increase energy levels in certain parts of the spectrum while reducing it in others.

Reflected solar radiation will take on the properties of the material that reflected it. It will be a highly modified solar radiation spectrum in general.

Atmospheric Filtering

The closer to the poles that you live, the more atmospheric filtering of solar radiation that takes place. This is due to the air mass being higher nearer to the poles. Let us see what 42 degrees latitude gives for air mass:

At summertime we have to subtract 23.5 degrees from the latitude for summer solstice:

Air mass =1/cos (42-23.5 degrees) = 1.05 air mass at summer.

In spring and fall we use the latitude of 42 degrees:

Air mass =1/cos (42 degrees) = 1.35 air mass at spring/fall

Now let's add in 23.5 degrees to the equation for winter solstice:

Air mass = 1/cos (42+23.5 degrees) = 2.41 air mass in winter

As we can see, air mass increases significantly in winter time. Winter has a 2.29 increase in air mass when compared to the summer, it more than doubles. Seasonal affect disorder syndrome (SADS) appears to be global position dependent with almost none at the equator and increases to a high prevalence near to the poles. It appears to be the atmospheric filtering of the solar radiation that causes seasonal affect disorder syndrome (SADS).

Given the large number of people who appear to be affected during wintertime in these locations nearer to the poles, we can assume that there is something going on regarding human health in these locations.

It is possible that the atmospheric pollution has made some of these locations optically toxic to humans during wintertime.

The effect is much worse the closer you get to the poles, as the air mass increases. At the poles it can be at the maximum value of approximately 38 all day long. If the solar radiation is toxic at this air mass, you would not want to be in this location.

Speed of Light

The speed of light is regarded as 186,282 miles per hour in a vacuum. The interesting thing about the speed of light is that it slows down when it passes through any type of gas, liquid or solid. Of particular note is the speed at which it passes through glass.

1,260 hundred miles per hour is the approximate speed of light through glass.

The refractive index is a measure how the speed of light is affected as it passes through a material. Glass has a refractive index of about 1.5, depending on the glass.

The formula for the refractive index is:

Refractive index = speed of light / speed of light through material

Solar Radiation & Weather

The strength of the Sun at ground level is dependent on the weather. The main factors that affect the Suns strength are clouds, snow, shade and latitude. Let us now explore the effects of the weather in more detail:

Irradiance

Irradiance is a measure of how much sunlight the Sun is producing at ground level. It is given in watts per meter squared or W/m^2. This value can range from $0W/m^2$ at night through to over $1,500W/m^2$ during a day interspersed with large fluffy clouds. This value of $1,500W/m^2$ is larger than what you would receive in Space. The reason why we can get greater values at ground level is due to what is known as the "Cloud Effect". Normally the sunlight is traveling in a straight line from the Sun to the ground with some atmospheric scattering. However, when clouds are present they can also reflect and can act like lenses to send some extra sunlight to the ground. This effect can be a few minutes long in duration when it occurs. The diagrams on the following pages demonstrates the "cloud effect" as applied to a solar module.

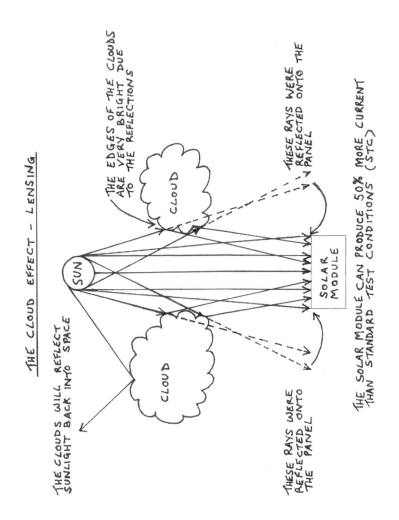

THE CLOUD EFFECT - LENSING

THE EDGES OF THE CLOUDS ARE VERY BRIGHT DUE TO THE REFLECTIONS

THESE RAYS WERE REFLECTED ONTO THE PANEL

THE CLOUDS WILL REFLECT SUNLIGHT BACK INTO SPACE

CLOUD

CLOUD

SUN

SOLAR MODULE

THESE RAYS WERE REFLECTED ONTO THE PANEL

THE SOLAR MODULE CAN PRODUCE 50% MORE CURRENT THAN STANDARD TEST CONDITIONS (STC)

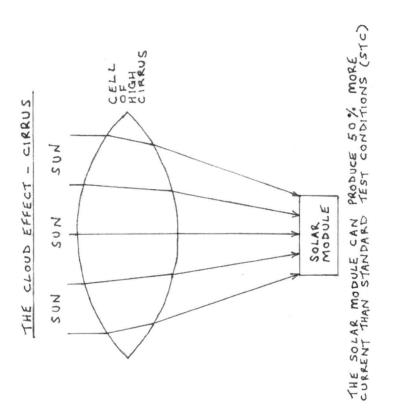

THE CLOUD EFFECT - CIRRUS

CELL OF HIGH CIRRUS

SUN SUN SUN SUN

SOLAR MODULE

THE SOLAR MODULE CAN PRODUCE 50% MORE CURRENT THAN STANDARD TEST CONDITIONS (STC)

Other effects on irradiance are the snow effect, the water effect (lake/ocean/wet surfaces after rain), the building effect and albedo. Snow cover, water, glass covered buildings, reflective painted buildings and roofs, and the albedo of the area surrounding the human environment can reflect extra sunlight into it. Each effect can produce an increase in power. If you find yourself having to wear sunglasses in your environment for your eyes to be comfortable, then you probably have light reflections taking place.

Air Mass

Air mass is a measurement of the the amount of atmosphere that the sunlight has to pass through to get to the ground. It varies with the seasons and also the location on the earth. Within the tropics, air mass will reach its maximum power value of 1 during summertime. Air mass 1 corresponds to the Sun being directly overhead, air mass increases as the Sun moves from directly overhead down to the horizon. At the horizon the air mass is approximately 38.

Locations that are at or near air mass 1 in summertime in the USA are all Hawaiian islands, Florida and Texas. In summertime the air mass will move closer to 1 in the continental USA.

Clouds

Clouds come in many forms. An important question is how do clouds affect solar irradiance? The list below will help with understanding the effects of clouds on solar irradiance at air mass 1 (solar noon within the tropics in summertime):

- Clear, sunny skies will give approximately 1,130W/m^2. The transmission characteristics of the atmosphere will vary in clear skies, sometimes being relatively transparent and other times being more opaque and this affects irradiance values. Air quality is a major factor for the transmission of sunlight through the atmosphere. Particulate matter in the atmosphere will reduce the transmission level and may cause interference effects.

- Thin cirrus will give approximately 1,000W/m^2. Thin cirrus will give even and relatively stable irradiance levels due to scattering of the light.

- Thick cirrus will give approximately 750W/m^2.

- Thin clouds will give about 500W/m^2.

- Thick clouds will give about 250W/m^2. No shadows on the ground will be present

- Thick clouds with a visibly dark sky will give about 100W/m^2. No shadows on the ground will be present. You will not be able to see the location of the Sun in the sky.

- Broken clouds will give surges of about $1,500W/m^2$ and reductions to about $100W/m^2$ of irradiance due to the cloud effect. The rate and length of time for these surges and reductions is dependent on the speed of the clouds passing in front of the Sun.

Shade

Shade significantly reduces the solar radiation levels in the human environment. The best form of shade is that from nature, such as trees. The optimum solar environment for the human is under the tree canopy in the shade.

Altitude

A higher altitude location will increase the amount of solar radiation in the human environment, due to less scattering and absorption of the sunlight by the atmosphere. It also acts as a natural cooler. Generally a high altitude location will have a higher percentage of clearer skies during a year.

Snow and Ice

The reflection from the snow and ice will increase the solar radiation in winter time. The highest annual solar radiation power levels may occur in this environment.

Seasons

We have four distinct seasons of winter, spring, summer and autumn. We can word this another way as winter solstice (December 21), spring equinox (March 20), summer solstice (June 21) and autumn equinox (September 22). What does this mean to solar radiation power levels?

- The length of the day
- The angle of the sun (air mass)
- Heating and cooling
- Foliage
- Clouds
- Rain
- Hail
- Snow
- Albedo

Winter solstice is the shortest day of the year and summer solstice is the longest day of the year. Spring and autumn equinoxes are when day time is the same length of time as night time.

Regarding the angle of the Sun in the USA, winter solstice is when the Sun is at the lowest in the sky, or 23.5 degrees below the equator and summer solstice is when it is 23.5 degrees above the equator. Spring and autumn equinoxes are when the Sun is directly overhead at solar noon at the equator.

The changing seasons will affect rainfall and rain will cause the albedo to change during the year. A barren snow covered field will be a lot different to one filled with corn or flowers.

Climate Change

The Earth's weather system is highly complicated and we struggle to predict how it will behave. Massive localized flooding has started to become commonplace in human society. Historic weather records are commonly being broken. It's not just high temperatures, but seasonal snow patterns, cold weather temperatures and strange changes in the seasons. The glaciers are receding and the ice caps at the poles are melting at alarming rates.

Changing the composition of the atmospheric gasses is a strong possibility for causing these changes.

It is a scary thought that we are adding large amounts of trapped exhaust gasses into the air that we breathe through the use of fossil fuels and industrial processes. The biomass that created the gas, coal and oil may have developed in a different atmosphere and may have had a different gas composition to the atmosphere that developed in harmony with the humans. Adding these trapped exhaust gasses into our current atmosphere may be like pouring poison into the human air supply.

Climate change is very real and poses an extremely serious threat to mankind.

The book "The Weather of the Future: Heat Waves, Extreme Storms, and Other Scenes from a Climate-Changed Planet" by Heidi Cullen gives an insight of what could be heading our way.

High Cirrus

High cirrus may be a relatively new phenomenon. Old paintings of high cirrus do not seem to be prevalent. It is a common view in the sky today.

High cirrus may be a result of the following:

- Development of industry
- Development of cars
- Development of air travel
- Development of refrigeration and air conditioning
- Development and use of chemicals
- The massive release of trapped water vapor into the atmosphere
- The massive release of previously trapped gasses into the atmosphere

If high cirrus is a modern development, then we have to ask ourselves how serious is this? Research into ground based solar radiation indicates that high cirrus raises the ground based solar radiation levels at times. High levels of solar radiation may be able to induce disease into the human body.

Earthquake Light

Earthquake light is being reported around the world. Earthquake light appears to precede large earthquakes in the world. It appears as rainbow effects in the clouds and many people report strange cloud formations.

What could be causing this effect to occur?

First, we need to understand what sunlight is. Sunlight is solar radiation that originated at the largest nuclear reactor in the solar system, called the Sun. Solar radiation contains many types of frequencies of radiation and is classed as broad spectrum radiation. Solar radiation is energy.

There are a number of things that are definite about the atmosphere:

- It is polluted
- The pollution is acting like a filter
- There are many more molecules in it
- The solar radiation transmission has changed
- The clouds have changed

So what could be causing vivid colors in the sky? It is most likely pollution condensing out from gas to liquid form in the atmosphere. Have you ever noticed that oil and water when mixed together makes color effects like that of rainbows? It appears that air and pollution may do the same trick. Vivid colors are characteristic of the light interference effects that fossil fuels can produce.

So what about the earthquake effects? Could these be true? Perhaps. Solar radiation has an energy content of 1,366 W/m^2 in Space. So to get the next concept you need to adjust your thinking to that of energy. The earthquake effect is associated with strange colors in the sky. This appears to be a result of interference.

Interferometry is the study of light interference. Now, we know that solar radiation is energy and that the energy waves are interfering with each other. This produces what is known as constructive and deconstructive interference. So the pollution is causing energy interference, so it may produce radio waves, right? And it appears that it does, low frequency radio waves between 10 kHz and 20kHz are commonly reported at the same time of the observations of earthquake light.

So how much energy interference could it produce? It's hard to say, but large scale interference over an area of 10 square kilometers could produce up to 13.66 gigawatts of energy interference if all of the energy was converted!

$$10km^2 \times 1,000,000m^2 \times 1,366W/m^2 = 13,660,000,000W$$

An area of 10,000 square kilometers could potentially produce 13.66 terawatts of energy interference!

$$10,000km^2 \times 1,000,000m^2 \times 1,366W/m^2 = 13,660,000,000,000W$$

Most power stations are producing about 1 gigawatt of energy. That makes this equivalent to 13,660 power stations of energy production. It is a lot of energy!

So where is all of the energy going to go? Probably into the core of the Earth. Unfortunately, on its way there it will pass through the human environment and it is currently unknown if this presents a problem to the core or to the surface environment and the life there.

Earthquake light is an unproven, but currently plausible, effect in nature.

The theory presented here is known as the "Atmospheric Energy Interference" effect.

Toxic Light © Steven Magee

Possible Interference Cloud Formation

Holes in the clouds may cause interference effects.

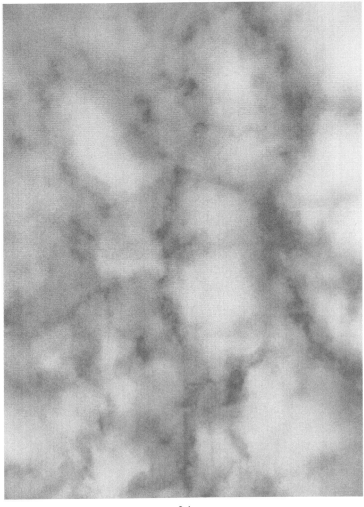

Colors in Clouds

Colors in clouds may be interference effects.

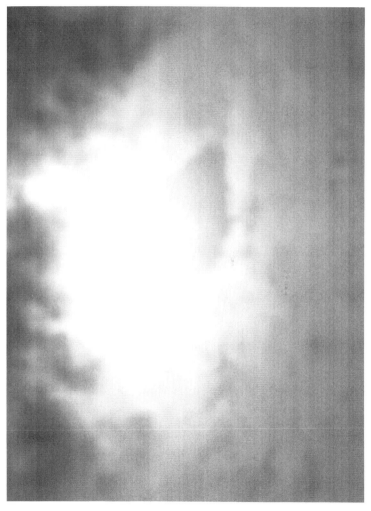

Albedo

Albedo is the Siamese twin of the cloud effect. They go everywhere together. Make sure that you are considering both effects when estimating solar radiation power levels. Albedo is the reflectivity of surfaces. A very well known effect in the world of astronomy.

Everything reflects light, even matt black surfaces reflect some low level of light, that's how we can see it. Everything our eyes can see is created from reflected light from surfaces. If your eyes can see these things, so can the rest of your body. If you need to put on your sunglasses, think about the reflection effects that may cause your eyes to be uncomfortable. Your body will sense the increase of solar radiation power levels as heat and you may start to sweat as your body warms up. You will need to identify these effects as it may be able to impact your health.

You should get used to assessing your environment for these albedo effects and start to avoid them if possible. Nature suppresses solar radiation for a reason. These albedo effects will probably put your body into an environment that it was never designed to cope with and the long term effects may be undesirable. The short term effect will be sunburn and possibly heatstroke.

Here is a list from Wikipedia that shows the albedo in various objects:

Object	Albedo
Fresh asphalt	0.04
Worn asphalt	0.12
Conifer forest	0.08 to 0.15
Deciduous trees	0.15 to 0.18
Bare soil	0.17
Green grass	0.25
Desert sand	0.4
New concrete	0.55
Ocean Ice	0.5–0.7
Fresh snow	0.80–0.90

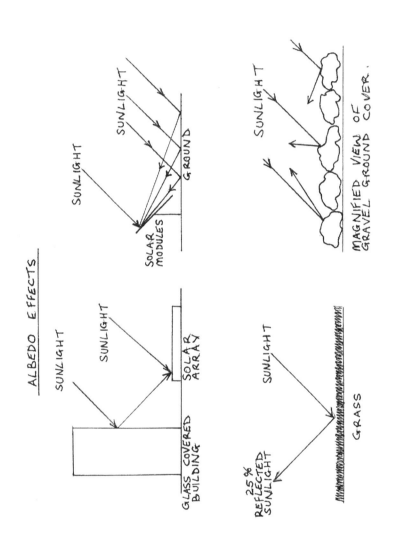

Toxic Light

Potentially toxic light is almost everywhere in modern society:

- Artificial Street lighting
- Artificial Home lighting
- Artificial Office lighting
- Anywhere where there is glass
- In your car
- In your home
- In your office
- Televisions of every type
- Computer monitors of every type
- At sunrise
- At sunset
- Near the north and south poles
- In any large city
- In chemical trails from aircraft
- In polluted atmosphere
- Anywhere where the tree canopy is not present

Toxic Light © Steven Magee

So what may toxic light be shown to do in the future? In the future the following conditions may be proven to be related to toxic light:

- Cancer
- Depression
- Heart attacks
- Circulation issues
- Diabetes
- Brain and nerve issues
- Disruption of circadian rhythm
- General aches and pains
- Aggression
- Psychiatric problems
- Almost any of the current medical problems in society may be related to toxic light

So your health and that of your family and children is important to you, so what can you do about this? The answer is quite simple:

- Move to the tropics, preferably the equator
- Live in an environment that has a tree canopy
- Eat fresh nourishing food that is grown in a natural way.

Toxic Light © Steven Magee

- Drink the water from the streams
- Don't live near to a city
- Avoid anything that is unnatural
- Avoid man-made materials, especially ones derived from fossil fuels

Aircraft Chemical Trails

The Sun as viewed through an aircraft chemical trail. Chemical trails of all types may cause toxic light.

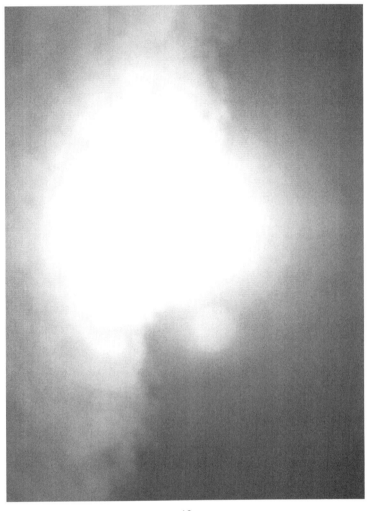

Man-Made Reflections

Man-made solar reflections have raised the solar radiation levels in society. These occur from many sources and we will list some of them here:

- Light colored paints
- Glossy paints
- Smooth engineered surfaces
- Glass
- Mirrors
- Reflective glass
- Roofing materials
- Cars and transportation systems
- Tall structures

There are many sources of man-made reflections and you should become accustomed to assessing your optical environment. Learn to identify these reflective items and assess their impact on solar radiation.

We will now look into what you will find in a modern man-made environment.

Toxic Light © Steven Magee

<u>High Solar Radiation</u>

We are constantly walking around in an energy field of
broad spectrum solar radiation that originated at the
largest nuclear reactor in the solar system, called the Sun.
It is important that this energy level be kept low for
human health. The trees and plants, also known as nature,
provide this function and aid human health.

You should avoid watching the sunrises and sunsets
regularly due to the filtered nature of the solar radiation.
It is this filtering that generates the amazing colors.
Unfortunately, staring at the Sun during this time appears
to be bad for human health. It may have the potential to
make you ill through solar radiation induced disease if it
becomes a regular habit.

General exposure to the direct view of the Sun delivers a
lot of energy to your body and this can be felt as heat and
also sensed by the eyes as brightness and you will need to
wear sunglasses due to this. There are no doubts that the
Sun is a carcinogen and it is wise to avoid direct views of
it.

Glass rooms, such as conservatories, should be avoided.
They are generally full of reflections and these boost the
radiation levels inside them. If you have one of these
rooms, you would be wise to fill it with plant life in order
to reduce the solar radiation levels inside it.

East, South and West facing windows let in a lot of direct solar radiation. You should not spend time too close to windows in this orientation. Natural window coverings are recommended. Plants should be placed next to windows like this. Desks should not be placed under these windows.

As for your eyes, ultraviolet (UV) rated sunglasses should be worn when the solar radiation levels are unnaturally high and these should be of an appropriate level of black tint. Mirrored, colored or polarized lenses should be avoided due to the modification of the solar radiation that takes place with these. You should view the light that your eyes receive as a nutrient and you want to keep it as natural as possible.

Environment

Humans have developed modern engineering materials that appear at times to increase the solar radiation levels in the human environment.

Increased levels of solar radiation are a concern due to the Sun being the largest nuclear reactor in the solar system. The nuclear energy that is received by the Earth has limited filtering by the Earth's atmosphere and the distance from the Sun. The human body is adapted to work well in a natural environment that has natural levels of solar radiation in it.

If the natural environment is changed and the solar radiation levels become unnatural, then it may cause illness and disease in humans. It may also affect the Earth on a global scale if the change is large enough.

It is important as humans progress and become more knowledgeable that we relate our progression to where we originated from and catalog the observed changes in the health of humans. When large numbers of humans are displaying health issues, it may be an indication that we have progressed in the wrong direction.

Mistakes are natural in human progression. Indeed, many mistakes are normal on the path to eventual success in society. It may be time to review where we are today as humans and to see if mistakes have been made and if a change in direction is now needed in order to chart the path to a healthy human society.

The environment is a complex interaction of many variables and working from the top down, some of these are:

- The Sun
- The Moon
- The Moon's orbit
- The Earth's orbit
- Space solar radiation
- Layers of different atmosphere
- Layers of different clouds
- Layers of increasing pressures
- Layers of different temperatures
- Atmospheric water vapor content
- Precipitation
- Atmospheric gas content
- Tree canopy
- Reflectivity of the solar radiation/tree canopy interface
- Ground level air pressure

- Ground level gasses
- Ground level temperature
- Ground level solar radiation
- Ground vegetation
- Reflectivity of the solar radiation/ground interface
- Temperature difference at the air/ground interface
- Seasonal fertilization
- Soil quality and water content
- Layers of different underground systems
- Water table
- Trapped biomass from past worlds
- Heat layers
- Pressure layers
- Molten core

Regarding bodies of water, we have also:

- Temperature of the air at the air/water interface
- Air pressure at the air/water interface
- Gasses at the air/water interface
- Temperature difference at the air/water interface
- Reflectivity of the air/water interface
- Water quality at the air/water interface

- Water temperature at the air/water interface
- Waves
- Water currents
- Chemical content of the water
- Layers of different water types
- Pressure layers

All function together to create the atmosphere that we live in. Probably the biggest things that will affect the human environment are:

- Solar radiation levels
- Solar radiation reflections
- Tree canopy
- Vegetation environment
- Air quality
- Air temperature
- Water vapor content of the air
- Precipitation

Let us now take a look at some of these factors and see what is happening with them.

Trees

Trees are made predominantly from air. The tree absorbs the air as it grows and converts it into a solid. The air is converted into wood and leaves. Trees trap large amounts of carbon dioxide through this process. It only occurs during the growth process.

Trees are composed of approximately 50% carbon and 50% water. This is where their mass comes from. Trees extract carbon from the air for their growth. The carbon dioxide levels in the atmosphere go down during spring and summer as the carbon is extracted for leaf growth. In the autumn and winter it increases again as the trees drop the leaves and they are broken down through composting.

Modern human society has cut down a significant number of trees to allow the land to be farmed for agriculture use. The removal of these trees released the trapped carbon and water back into the environment and may have changed the atmospheric water and carbon dioxide content of the planet.

Have you noticed that new growth on trees is a much lighter green than the full grown leaves and stems? This appears to be due to a higher level of reflectivity of the new shoots. It appears that young growth on trees needs to absorb less solar radiation for a reason. It is quite possible that new growth would be damaged if it was absorbing the same levels of radiation as the older growth.

Trees absorb the majority of solar radiation that hits them. In environments where the trees have been removed, the solar radiation levels at ground level generally have significantly increased. This will result in increased heating of the ground and the surrounding air. It should come as no surprise that historic high temperature records appear to keep on being broken and it seems to be as a result of this.

The increased reflectivity of the ground means that more of the Suns energy is lost by being reflected back into Space. This should produce a net loss of energy received from the Sun by the Earth when compared to the past.

A hotter ground-level environment, higher ground-level solar radiation and higher air temperatures with lower energy absorption by the Earth appears to be the result currently.

Trees are a very efficient solar radiation absorber and humans would be foolish to ignore the effect of global tree reduction on the Earth's environment. Their conversion of solar radiation into different forms of energy appears to be needed to keep the environment in balance. They also appear to maintain a healthy solar radiation environment for humans.

Trees have a high level of absorption of water during rains. Most theories on water absorption by the planet relate to the soil acting like a sponge. The trees appear to exhibit the sponge action too. Trees appear to have the capacity to store large amounts of water and to slowly release it through evaporation.

Evaporation is how air conditioners work. Have you ever noticed that it is cooler when under a tree? That is evaporation combined with a lower solar radiation environment at work. Yes, trees work as natural air conditioners and solar radiation suppressors!

Trees appear to have a major function in the regulation of the global environment. Most people relate trees to the regulation of gasses in the atmosphere. Trees also appear to have a major function in the regulation of solar radiation absorption, water vapor in the atmosphere and water absorption by the Earth and this aspect of trees requires further study.

So why did we cut them down and pave our human environment with man made materials? I'm really not sure, you will have to ask the architects and city planners that question. It appears to have been a mistake.

To sum up, trees provide the following functions:

- Trap carbon through growth

- Absorb almost all solar radiation
- Convert a small amount of solar radiation to a different broad spectrum of scattered solar radiation
- Prevent solar radiation reflections
- Convert solar radiation energy into different forms of energy
- Provide the correct solar radiation environment for humans
- Create interference solar radiation
- Regulate the ground level solar radiation environment
- Fertilize the ground around them by dropping their leaves in autumn
- Cool the local environment
- Provide shade
- Provide regulation of gasses to the atmosphere
- Trap water
- Provide water absorption during rains
- Help prevent flooding during rains
- Provide water vapor regulation to the atmosphere

Plant Health

Plants are affected by many factors. Climate change is changing rainfall, humidity, air composition, solar radiation, heating and cooling. Plants are sensitive to any of these factors. When all of the factors start to change at once, it may lead to devastation in the plant world.

Seeds only germinate in a narrow range of temperatures. If the temperature changes and is outside of this range then germination will not occur.

Seeds will only germinate when there is sufficient light passing through the tree canopy. It appears that nature automatically fills holes in the tree canopy.

Seeds need a certain level of water to germinate. If this water level changes then they may not germinate.

Plants that appear to be well suited to constantly high levels of solar radiation appear to be those of the cactus family. They also have the ability to tolerate extremely low rainfall levels. Some of the plants in these desert environments appear to have the ability to move their leaves to match the level of solar radiation. When it is very high, they close them together and when it is low, they open their leaves to the Sun.

Plant leaves change with different solar radiation levels. The same plant will change the color, shape and size of the leaves to match the level of solar radiation that it receives. There is a limit to how adaptable each plant is and if the radiation gets outside of its range, the plant will start to show stress and depression symptoms and may eventually die.

A changed radiation environment for plants may have the following effects:

- Leaf changes
- Growth changes
- Accelerated growth
- Stress
- Reproduction issues
- Depression
- Death

Loss of many varieties of plants may cascade down the food chain to the humans. As the plants die off, the life support system for humans will start to reduce and human starvation may result.

Plant life is like the canary in the cage. When it starts to die off, we know we have problems. To ignore plant die off would be like the human race committing suicide. Human extinction would surely follow.

Open Fields

The trees were removed to make way for the open fields that we now have to grow the crops needed to support the humans in the cities. The open crop fields are generally not natural, they are engineered by humans.

Open fields that are not planted and are just dirt will absorb solar radiation energy. This will heat the soil which in turn will transfer that heat to the air above it.

Open fields of soil or crops generally have a much higher reflectivity than trees. This effect can be seen from airplanes and satellite images. This means that less solar energy is absorbed by the field compared to a forest. A net solar energy loss occurs due to the field reflecting solar energy back into the atmosphere and some of that solar energy ends up returning into space.

The reflected solar energy that does not make it back into space ends up being absorbed by the atmosphere. This is an extra addition of energy to the atmosphere that should appear as an air temperature increase.

It sounds a lot like global warming.

We should probably be growing crops in the shade of native trees. Some types of crops that are not grown in the shade of trees may end up with a level of solar poisoning in them from excessive solar radiation exposure. It would be undesirable for humans to eat such food.

The solar poisoning effect may also exist in meat and fish that are farmed using modern agricultural techniques. It may be important to grow these foods in natural environments that provide natural shade cover.

Fossil Fuels

Fossil fuels are widely used throughout the world. The easy fuels have been accessed and depleted. Now we are developing the more difficult sources of these fuels with the associated increased risks that this creates.

We are told that these fuels have been trapped in the Earth and have formed from decayed matter that existed millions of years ago. As we have discussed, the forests form by converting carbon dioxide and water into wood and leaves. These have now converted into trapped natural gas, coal and oil.

When we drill into the Earth and bring the trapped coal, gas and oil to the surface, it is burned and releases the exhaust gasses from it into the atmosphere. These add to the composition of the atmosphere. The important concept here is "add". No one really understands how adding large amounts of exhaust gasses into a stable atmosphere affects it. It is a mystery.

The atmosphere is a really thin layer on the surface of the Earth. To add large amounts of trapped exhaust gasses to it is like gambling with our future. If the gamble does not work out well, the effects could be serious and may not be able to be undone.

The extraction and burning of fossil fuels is strongly linked to climate change. Humans are adding large amounts of exhaust gasses to an atmosphere that took millions of years to develop in harmony with humans. It may reach a critical point in the future where the human body can not keep pace with the changing composition of the atmosphere. This will place the human body under continual stress and may push it into a diseased state and onto premature death.

We have already witnessed the effect of a poisonous local atmosphere with the human habit of smoking. A poisonous global atmosphere may eventually lead to widespread human disease and onto a possible human extinction. If this happens, nature will take over and reforest the planet, restoring the balance once again and another less invasive species will become dominant.

The problem with adding lots of extra molecules to a stable atmosphere is that it may create interference of the solar radiation transmission from Space to the surface of the Earth. If this happens, then it may increase the illness and disease rates in humans. In some parts of the world, solar radiation interference may already be occurring.

So what exactly are fossil fuels? The correct answer is that no one really knows. They may not even be made from fossils. The correct name for these fuels is "substances from unknown origin". They are toxic to humans. Abiogenic and abiotic are terms that can be used to describe these fuels. Their meaning is "without life".

The fossil fuel industry has created the biggest threat to human extinction and the extinction of the majority of the Earth's animal and plant species and they have done this in a period of just over 100 years.

There is massive pollution entering the atmosphere on a daily basis and it is becoming more toxic, to the point that it appears to be harming mankind. Fossil fuel use should be stopped as we know it is toxic to humanity.

Pollution

Pollution comes in many forms and some of these are:

- Unnaturally high levels of solar radiation
- Unnaturally low levels of solar radiation
- Unnaturally filtered solar radiation
- Interference solar radiation
- Man-made light sources
- Extraction and burning of fossil fuels
- Industrial processes
- Chemicals
- Nuclear technologies
- Mining

Unnatural levels of solar radiation should be expected to induce illness and disease into almost everything. The human, animal, plant and marine kingdoms will all be greatly affected. Unfortunately, the unnatural levels of solar radiation in today's modern society appear to be man-made.

So how can it be prevented? Simply by stopping all man-made emissions into the atmosphere, rivers and oceans.

Toxic Light © Steven Magee

Rapid reforestation of the planet with trees would essentially restore the lungs of the Earth and start to trap the man-made emissions that are present in the atmosphere.

Just like humans, the planet has two lungs. The other is the ocean. The pollution into the ocean needs to stop so that the ocean can recover and restore its lung capacity.

Sunlight is regarded as having the color of white. It is quite possible that thousands of years ago the sunrises and sunsets were white, not the reds and oranges that we have today. White is regarded a pure. Unfiltered sunlight matches this color.

It is recommended that we move as quickly as we can back to an atmosphere that does not excessively filter the sunlight and change its color. This appears to be required for humanity to return to a healthy society.

By stopping pollution today, we can start creating the world that our children can thrive in. If we don't make these changes quickly, then there may be no future for our children. Humanity will most likely go extinct.

So how can we gauge the progression of air pollution? The answer turns out to be relatively easy. Humans have been painting sunsets and moon-sets for hundreds of years in their artwork. Fortunately, much of this artwork has been kept in pristine condition and is available to view.

When reviewing the artwork of sunsets and moon-sets, we see that the orange/red sunset appears to be a relatively modern phenomenon. Prior to this, sunsets did not appear to be orange/red. They were relatively white.

Evidence of atmospheric pollution will be at its worst when the Sun or the Moon is near to the horizon. This is due to the radiation from these objects passing through the thickest part of the atmosphere. This is called high air mass in the scientific community. The radiation is subjected to the most atmospheric filtration at this time. Air mass is 1 when the sun is at zenith and down at the horizon it is near to 38. This means that the solar radiation receives approximately 38 times more atmospheric filtration at sunset.

Pollution causes the visible light to turn orange/red due to the filtering effects of pollution on this light. The more pollution there is, the redder it will look. This can be seen on the island of Hawaii where the Kilauea volcano is erupting and pumping out gasses into the environment. The sunsets on this island are red, like the color of blood.

This is a problem near the poles, due to the Sun being lower in the sky. The sunlight is subjected to much more filtration by the atmosphere for much longer periods of time. This may be unhealthy for people who live nearer to the poles.

Filtering solar radiation with pollution is probably a bad idea.

A good example of pollution in the atmosphere is on the cover of my first book "Solar Photovoltaic Design for Residential, Commercial and Utility Systems". This picture was taken from the summit of Kitt Peak National Observatory in Sells, Arizona, USA. At an elevation of approximately 6,875 feet, we can see a deep orange sunset. This sunset several hundred years ago probably would have been a white sunset. Orange and red sunsets are characteristic of a polluted atmosphere. Viewing the midday Sun through smoke also produces an orange or red view of it.

It is interesting that smoking causes cancer. Could it be that smokers are having cancer induced into them by the same effects as pollution creates with solar radiation?

Atmospheric Pollution

Atmospheric pollution can cause Sun filtering, polarization, diffraction and interference effects.

Tall Buildings

We saw in "Solar Reflections for Architects, Engineers and Human Health" that tall buildings appear to have the potential to raise the radiation levels on the outside of them. But what about the inside of them?

Tall buildings may be an issue to human health on a number of fronts. When you are on the upper floors and have a clear view of the world, everything around you also has a clear view of you too! This includes:

- Solar radiation
- Radiation reflections
- Wireless radiation

All types of radiation are more powerful with a direct line of sight to their source.

If you live in one of these buildings, it is recommended that you block the view with live plant life. They will absorb and modify the radiation levels for you. You should think of plant life as your guardian angel. They should make you feel good and, if you have flowers, they will look really pretty.

Structure Radiation

Structures appear to have the ability to modify the solar radiation by creating :

- Unnaturally high levels
- Modified solar radiation spectrum
- Diffraction effects
- Interference effects
- Polarization

This includes:

- Buildings
- Power lines & poles
- Large structures
- Roofs visible from the ground
- Antennas
- Wind turbines
- Solar power systems
- Power stations
- Power transmission lines
- Domes

- Tall buildings
- Lampposts
- Bridges
- Dams
- Street signs
- Storage tanks
- Cranes
- Chemical plants
- Industrial buildings
- Pyramids

You should be careful around anything man-made that is taller than a single story home until more is known on the subject.

Tall structures can be a problem as they may reflect a lot of solar radiation to the ground around them. This effect increases as you get closer to them.

Many types of structures create these solar radiation effects and the above list is just a short sample of the structures that can do this.

You should try to avoid being near tall structures during the main solar radiation hours of the day. Particularly near solar noon these effects are at their maximum. If you work in one of these structures, you should try and stay inside during your work day to avoid passing through the higher levels of solar radiation that they may create around them.

It is plausible that the structures in your environment may be able to affect your health.

It is recommended that the construction of tall structures be avoided and that if a large structure is required that it be located below ground level, such as in an old surface mine.

If a large structure is built above ground, then it should probably be covered in plant growth.

Power transmission and distribution lines should be routed underground wherever possible.

It is an interesting observation that almost all pyramids in the world have been found abandoned. The pyramid structure generates high levels of horizontal solar radiation around it. The human eyes, organs and body appear not to be designed to deal with these increased horizontal reflections.

PYRAMID SOLAR RADIATION

PYRAMIDS THAT ARE NEAR TO EACHOTHER CREATE A MAZE OF SOLAR RADIATION REFLECTIONS. THIS WILL BOOST THE SOLAR RADIATION LEVELS TO VERY HIGH POWERS.

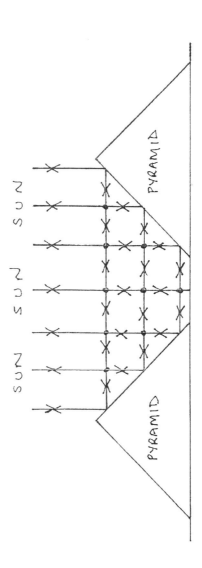

Toxic Light © Steven Magee

Pyramid Reflection

Pyramids can create horizontal solar radiation reflections.

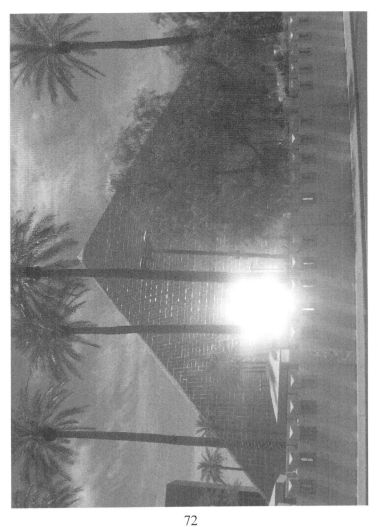

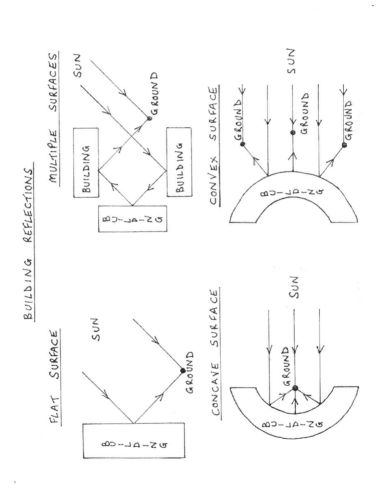

BUILDING REFLECTIONS

MULTIPLE SURFACES

FLAT SURFACE

CONVEX SURFACE

CONCAVE SURFACE

73

Building Acting as a Lens

The curved building acts as a lens to focus multiple Sun reflections to the same point. This is called the multiple-Sun effect.

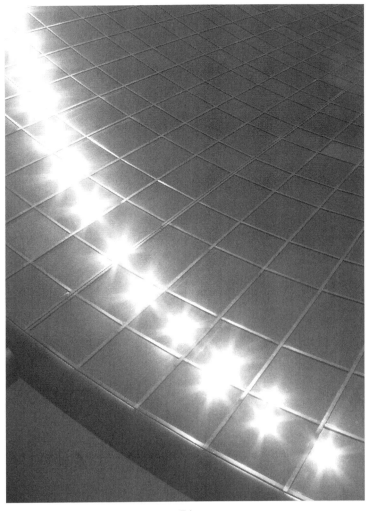

Toxic Light © Steven Magee

Power Pole Interference

The solar radiation distorts around the lines and poles and causes reflections, diffraction and interference effects.

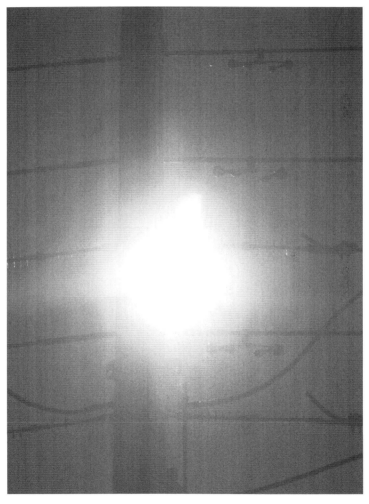

Lamppost Interference

The solar radiation bleeds into the lamppost and causes reflections, diffraction and interference effects.

Toxic Light © Steven Magee

Cell Phone Tower Interference

Towers and antennas may create reflections, diffraction and interference effects.

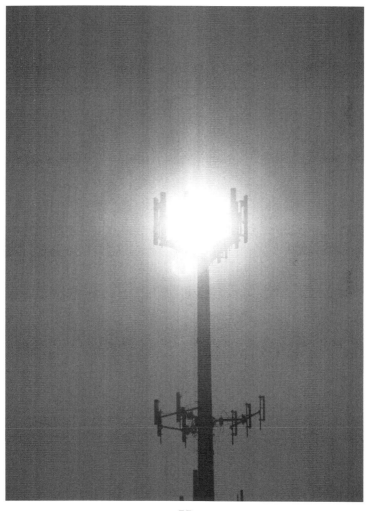

Alternate Energy

While alternate energy sources seem appealing, they have their problems too.

Solar Energy

Solar energy systems generally operate with low efficiencies and the solar radiation that is not converted into energy ends up either being reflected, diffracted, interfered with or turned into heat. They are all are undesirable. Heat may contribute to the effects of climate change. The reflections, diffraction and interference effects may raise the solar radiation levels around the systems to unnatural levels. Commercial and utility solar energy systems are essentially very large atmospheric plate heaters that cover extremely large areas of land. They may contribute to climate change rather than reduce it. The processes involved in making them may be toxic to the environment.

The book "Challenging the Chip: Labor Rights and Environmental Justice in the Global Electronics Industry" covers some of these production problems.

Wind Power

These systems are very large and tall. Tall structures may cause solar radiation reflections, diffraction and interference effects which are undesirable, as they may raise the radiation levels around them. They also kill flying animals, such as birds, insects and bats, as their blade tips can travel at approximately 250 miles per hour. If you examine a wind turbine blade, it may be covered in splattered bugs, just like the front of your car. The areas around wind turbines are becoming nature dead zones, due to:

- Air pressure waves that they create. People who live up to ten miles downwind of these turbines may complain about the noise that they can make.

- Wind turbines extract their energy from wind and affect the natural wind systems.

- Optically, they cause flicker to occur which the human body may be sensitive to. This may cause health problems in people who have a view of them.

- Vibrations in the ground around them

The book "The Wind Farm Scam" by John Etherington details some of these problems.

Tidal

Tidal systems disrupt the natural flow of water and may affect the underwater environment of the sea life.

Dams

These disrupt the natural flow of water and upset the life within the river. They create massive water evaporation into the atmosphere.

Wave

These systems have not been perfected yet and disrupt the natural flow of ocean water and ocean life.

Nuclear

Natural energy that has not been perfected. The mining and processing of the fuel is highly destructive to the environment. It generates a lot of waste heat, water evaporation and highly toxic waste that no one knows what to do with. The highly toxic waste will be around for thousands of years. The highly toxic waste is a disaster waiting to happen, as we have seen with the Fukushima nuclear disaster in Japan. Unfortunately, it appears that we may be leaving a highly poisonous discovery for a future generation that may not be aware of the dangers contained within the storage containers.

I'm not sure why we ever moved away from natural surface fuels. They are completely renewable. It is suggested that our dependance on energy be returned to natural bio-fuels, such as wood, at the earliest possible opportunity.

Humans are displaying an addiction to energy that appears to be like drug addiction. It rules their lives. Humans should be weaned off energy consumption in order to reduce this unnatural dependance that has been formed. If it continues then it may destroy the atmosphere and by association, lead to the extinction of humanity.

Houses should have trees placed around them to help keep them cool and reduce the air conditioning loads on the electrical grid. Ideally, houses should be located under the tree canopy due to the stable environmental conditions that it creates for humans.

The book "Sparking a Worldwide Energy Revolution" gives a good overview to the energy problems of today and possible ways forward.

The book "The False Promise of Green Energy" gives an overview of the green energy industry.

Glass

The use of glass for windows in homes is relatively modern. In past years glass was rougher and this can be seen in older buildings. The older glass appears to distort the images that pass through it and defects can be seen.

Float glass was later developed in the 1960's and is a very smooth engineered surface. Most modern glass is float glass.

With the advent of trying to be energy efficient, most glass now has coatings that affect the solar radiation transmission through it. On the outside of the glass, much of the solar radiation is reflected back into the environment, adding to the solar radiation levels there. Of the solar radiation that passes through the glass, it is now modified and unnatural. This type of glass started to appear in the late 1980's.

It is plausible that the glass in your environment may be able to affect your health.

It is recommended that all glass on the inside of a building have natural coverings placed in front of it to prevent reflections and also to diffuse the modified spectrum solar radiation that passes through it.

On the outside of the building, it is recommended that plants be placed in front of the glass to absorb the reflected solar radiation. On a tall building, the windows should be covered with non-reflective downward facing louvers that prevent solar radiation reflections.

You may want to avoid spending time next to windows and if you have a desk with a view, move it away from the window or reduce the solar radiation by using a window covering.

Conservatories have become popular house additions and these are generally made out of glass. Again, use window coverings and plants to reduce the solar radiation levels in these types of glass buildings.

Double and triple glazing may pose a problem due to the following effects:

- Distortion of the glass
- Chromatic aberrations
- Coated energy saving glass

The distorted glass occurs due to the slight vacuum that is present between the panes of glass. This may cause the reflected light to be lensed into a high powered beam of solar radiation. The power content of this may exceed that found in Space.

Chromatic aberrations may be an issue, due to the dispersion effect that it has on the spectrum of the light. This causes the light to be dispersed into the colors of the spectrum of the light and can be commonly seen on the surfaces where the light lands. It typically appears as a rainbow effect or a color at the edge of the light on the surface that it is cast on to.

Lead lights, window screens and dirt on the window pane may have the ability to cause diffraction and interference effects. It is unknown if any of these may be an issue to human health.

As you can see, we still have much to learn about the different types of glass and their interaction with human health.

The following pictures show how reflective double glazed glass can be and how it can randomly distort light.

Double Glazed Windows

These three identical windows are at the entrance to my house.

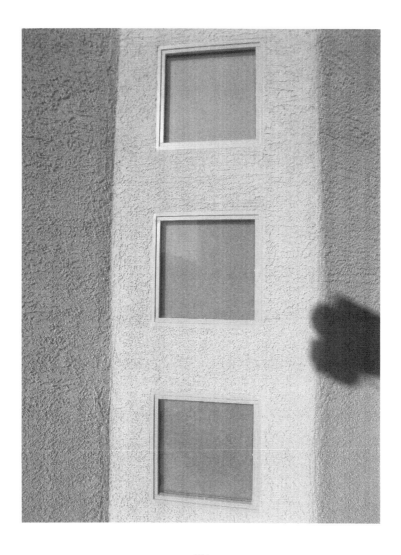

Double Glazed Reflections

These are the reflections that the double glazed glass creates when the Sun is reflected from them. As you can see, each reflection is unique which indicates that each pane of glass has a different type of distortion.

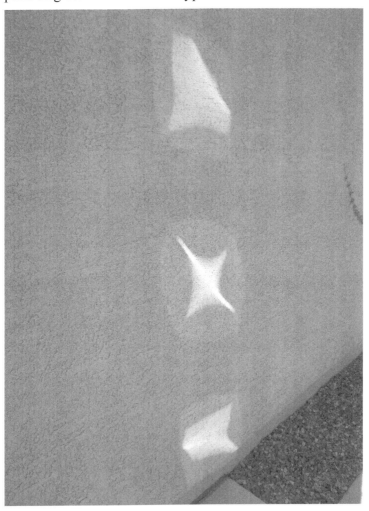

Privacy Glass

Privacy glass is commonly found in bathrooms and restrooms. It is glass that has patterns in it or has been intentionally produced with ripples in it. The problems with putting distortions into glass is that you affect how the light transmits through it.

Some light will pass through with relatively little change, whereas other light will be highly distorted. Around these types of windows you will generally find chromatic aberrations which will show up as colors on the edges of the bright patches of light that the window casts on the surrounding surfaces. Sometimes you will see rainbow effects with the glass spreading out the light into the color spectrum.

Bright and dark patches of light that textured windows create are a concern, as they can act like lenses and focus the light. These bright patches are high areas of solar radiation. Around windows that act like lenses you will commonly find these areas of high solar radiation and their effects on human health are currently unknown.

The following pictures show the effects that these windows create.

Heavily Textured Glass

This is the view through a glass block in my bathroom window. Note the heavy distortion in the image.

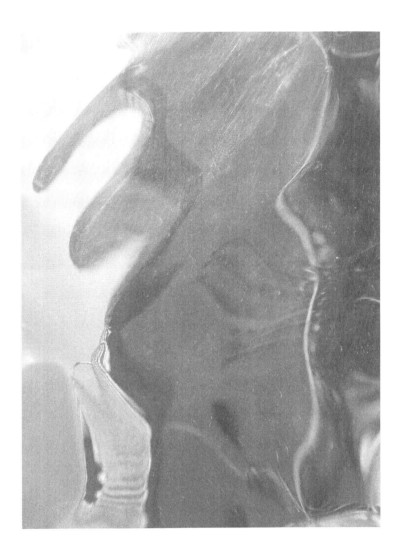

Chromatic Aberration

Chromatic aberration caused by the light transmission through the glass can cause colors to appear in the light that is cast onto surfaces. In this case, it created a rainbow effect.

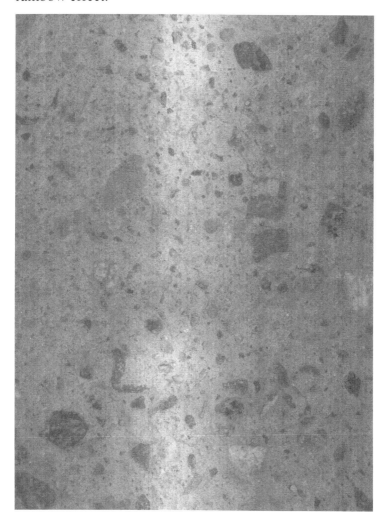

Chromatic Aberration

In this case the white light had a fringe of blue light at the top of the image that was caused by chromatic aberration.

Window Coatings

Anything unnatural that filters the broad spectrum of solar radiation will create an artificial and possibly toxic environment for humans.

Glass coatings modify the solar radiation spectrum on both the outside and inside of the glass. Many of these coatings cannot be seen by the human eye and the glass will appear to be transparent to optical light. The glass may be highly reflective to other wavelengths such as ultraviolet (UV), infrared (IR) or radio.

The atmosphere when mixed with pollution is just like a window coating. If you fill the atmosphere with toxins, then you really cannot be surprised if the solar radiation transmission through it becomes toxic to humans.

Sunscreens act like window coatings and modify the solar radiation received by the body. You should avoid the use of sunscreens, as they may be toxic to the body if used daily. The man-made chemicals may also have an ability to poison the body in the long term.

The following pictures are of coated double glazed glass.

Sun Refection in Double Glazed Glass

This is how the Sun looked when reflected from the double glazed pane of glass. There were three reflections of the Sun!

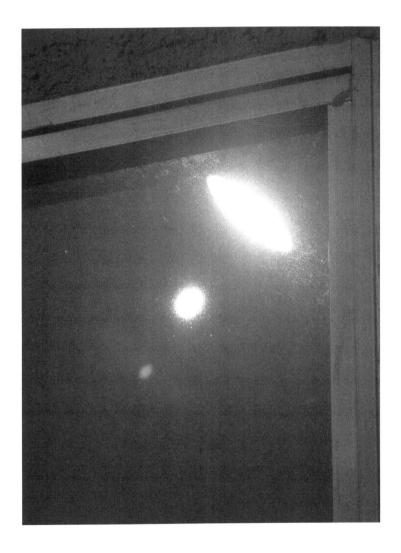

Wall Reflection

And this was the reflection from it onto the wall. Note the bright patches of solar radiation that are actually higher in power than that of Space!

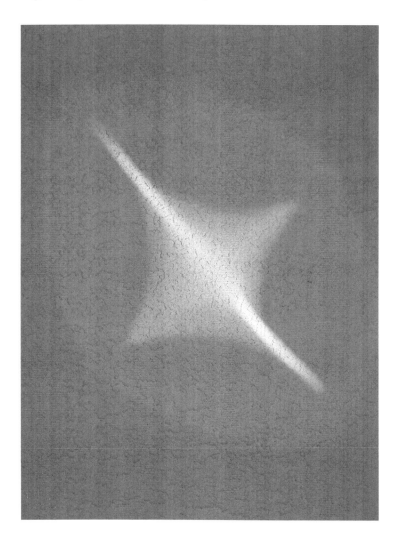

Roofs

Roofs that can be seen from the ground can reflect solar radiation to the ground and increase the solar radiation levels.

It is recommended that roofs that can be seen from the ground have trees placed near to them to reduce the solar radiation reflections that they create.

Roofs that absorb solar radiation will act like heaters and radiate their heat into the surrounding air. In a city environment, there are many buildings that will be heating the surrounding air and raising the city temperature.

Multiple houses that are situated on curves may act like lenses. They have the potential for the solar radiation that is reflected from their pitched roofs to combine and significantly raise the solar radiation levels around them. This is a concern to humans who may pass through these high solar radiation environments.

It is plausible that the roof on your house may be able to affect your health.

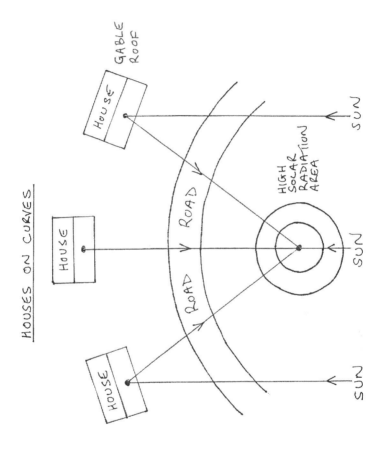

Air Conditioning

Air conditioners remove heat from the interior of buildings. This heat is formed by the absorption of solar radiation and hot outside air temperatures by the building. Air conditioners work by using energy to transfer the heat energy from the inside of the building to the outside. They essentially work by dumping large amounts of heat and energy into the outside air and raise the outside temperature.

It sounds a lot like global warming.

Air conditioning has allowed humans to live almost anywhere in the world. Without it, many population centers would not exist. Unfortunately, it has increased energy consumption significantly and a corresponding release of fossil fuel exhaust emissions into the atmosphere. Future human population increases should be focused on areas that have stable climates that do not require the use of air conditioners.

Paints

Modern paints have been developed that are highly reflective. These work by reflecting solar radiation that hits the paint back into the environment. This is undesirable from a human perspective as it raises the solar radiation levels around the building or structure.

It is plausible that the solar radiation that is reflected from the paint on the outside of your house may be able to affect your health.

Outdoor paints should be developed that reflect very low levels of solar radiation. It is suggested that they should mimic nature and have the same reflected solar radiation spectrums as trees and flowers. Gloss paints should be avoided and paints should have low levels of reflectivity.

Ground Materials

Solar radiation can be reflected up from the ground. The level of the reflection is dependent on the material that the ground is made of. A dry and smooth concrete sidewalk generally will reflect about 55% of the solar radiation back into the environment. It will have a modified solar radiation spectrum to match the material that reflected it.

The power of the reflection increases the closer you are to it, as such, the feet, ankles and knees are most vulnerable to these types of solar radiation reflections.

You should avoid using smooth man-made materials for ground cover. Instead, use rough natural materials such as wood or dark stone.

It is plausible that the ground materials may be able to affect your health.

Architecture

The multiple-Sun reflections do not seem to appear in nature. I have spent many weeks looking for them in the National Parks of the USA and failed to locate the multiple-Sun effect. The National Parks are as close to a natural environment that you will find in the USA.

Nature creates scattered, diffracted and interference sunlight at much lower power levels. This averages out to much lower irradiance values compared to those of the cities. There must be a reason why nature does this and it would be foolish to ignore nature.

Nature is in harmony with the Sun. We must look to nature and follow its guidance. Nature reflects light by scatttering, interfering with it and creating low power levels. We should do the same in our societies.

It is quite possible that we are supposed to receive the light that nature creates. Light from trees and grass may have beneficial effects on human health. Just ask any camper how they feel when they are camping in a natural environment. Generally they will tell you that they love the clean air. What they were not aware of is that the light is also very different in nature and they may be experiencing beneficial effects from this as well.

How can we mimic nature? Here are a few suggestions:

- Use rough surfaces throughout
- Use natural building materials such as rough stone and wood
- Use dark colors that absorb light
- Use colors that reflect light with the same color spectrum's that are found in nature.
- Sidewalks and roads should be made from rougher, less reflective materials
- Create shade wherever possible
- Plant more trees and create a natural environment
- Reflect only scattered light
- Shade reflective surfaces with non-reflective downward facing louvers
- Use flat roofs that can not be seen from the ground
- Limit the height of the buildings to that of the trees
- Keep to single story construction if possible

Architecture should be designed by architects who are trained in optics. They must understand the reflective effects of their construction materials. A good understanding of albedo is a must.

Engineers must understand that buildings and construction materials create parallel, semi-parallel, and non-parallel reflections, polarization, diffraction and interference effects, modified solar radiation and high levels of albedo, and they will need to factor that into their particular engineering field.

Human health in a multiple-Sun environment needs to be evaluated and understood by the medical profession. The long term effects of continual high irradiance exposure and modified solar radiation are currently unknown.

We are still constructing mirrored buildings. Perhaps it is time to take a break and examine the human solar radiation environment before committing to any more buildings like this?

Houses

The arrangement of houses can create concentrated solar radiation reflections from them. Multiple houses that are arranged in a curved formation can act like a lens and focus the solar radiation reflected from them into the surrounding area.

If you are feeling ill frequently, you should assess the solar radiation environment that the houses in your area create to rule this out. Pay close attention to headaches, nausea and head or facial nerve pains.

Multiple people dying before the age of seventy may be an indication of problems in a street. Look for the following history in residents:

- Brain tumors
- Strokes
- Brain and spinal cord problems
- Mental issues
- Nerve issues
- Heart attacks
- Cancer
- Learning difficulties in the young
- General health problems

It is plausible that your neighborhood may be able to affect your health.

Haunted houses may have their root cause in an unnatural solar radiation environment. This may show up as the people living there having strange dreams. An unnatural radiation environment may well cause hallucinations, giving the sensation of the house being haunted!

When purchasing a house it is recommended that you assess the solar radiation environment of both the house and the surrounding area.

House Selection

Here are some hints and tips for selecting low solar radiation homes:

- Avoid houses that:
    - Are on curves in the road due to lensing effects that the reflections from multiple houses may create
    - Are painted in light reflective colors
    - Have smooth exterior walls
    - Have lots of glass
    - Have pitched roofs that can be seen from the ground
    - Are paved with modern reflective construction materials
    - Are overlooked by taller structures
    - Have views of the roofs of the surrounding houses
    - Are near built up areas, especially industrial zones
    - Are devoid of natural wildlife
    - Have no trees or vegetation

- Look for houses that:
    - Are surrounded by trees

- Have plenty of vegetation
- Are covered in climbing plants
- In a natural setting
- Are single story only
- Are old and have aged
- Are made of natural rough materials such as wood and dark stone
- Are painted in dark non-reflective colors on the outside
- Have the majority of windows facing the Pole
- Have window coverings on both the inside and outside of the house
- Have bedrooms facing the Pole
- Have underground utilities

For information on healthy buildings, the free film "First Earth" at http://www.davidsheen.com/firstearth/film.htm provides excellent advice.

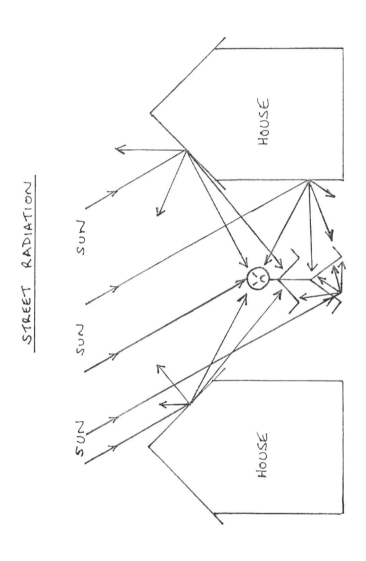

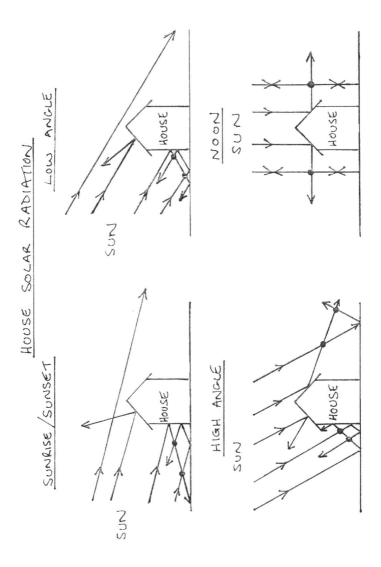

Cars

The prolific adoption of cars and transport systems has been rapid over the last few decades. Cars and transportation systems can be highly reflective. This increases the solar radiation levels in the environment.

Cars in particular create horizontal solar radiation reflections. You should keep them in the shade or in a garage to prevent this.

The face, neck, chest and reproduction areas are especially vulnerable to these solar radiation reflections, due to them being horizontal.

They also dump heat and exhaust gasses into their environment.

These effects are undesirable and humans should start to develop transportation systems that are either underground or shielded from view by vegetation and trees. Humans should move away from regular car commuting to and from work and into local working that is within walking distance.

It is plausible that cars may be able to affect your health.

Artificial Light

Artificial light sources are a concern as the light is different from sunlight. So you are worried about artificial lighting and are thinking that you can fix it by using full spectrum lighting products? Think again. While full spectrum lighting products sound appealing, the truth is that there is no such thing as full spectrum artificial lighting. It is a marketing ploy.

What full spectrum really means is that the light is as close to the Suns spectrum as can be possibly made using current technology. Unfortunately it is not sunlight and never will be.

All types of artificial lighting have the possibility of making you ill. Artificial lighting should be avoided if your health is important to you.

If you are going to have artificial lighting in your environment, then it should have a plant in front of it so that the light becomes modified by the plant. This is shown on the next page.

Light Modification by Plants

Here is the "Star of Bethlehem" as produced by a halogen lamp and a plant

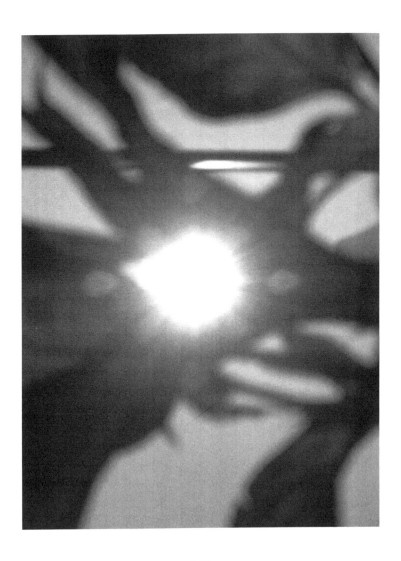

Color temperatures can be used to specify light sources. Here is a list of the color temperatures in kelvin of modern light sources, as listed on Wikipedia:

- 1,700K Match flame
- 1,850K Candle flame, sunset/sunrise
- 2,700–3,300K Incandescent light bulb
- 3,350K Studio "CP" light
- 3,400K Studio lamps, photofloods, etc.
- 4,100K Moonlight, xenon arc lamp
- 5,000K Horizon daylight
- 5,500–6,000K Vertical daylight, electronic flash
- 6,500K Daylight, overcast
- 9,300K CRT screen

As can be seen, the color temperature varies between the different sources and also the different times of the day.

The Color Rendering Index, or CRI for short, is similar to the color temperature. Wikipedia says the "Color rendering index, or CRI, is a measure of the quality of color light, devised by the International Commission on Illumination (CIE). It generally ranges from zero for a source like a low-pressure sodium vapor lamp, which is monochromatic, to one hundred, for a source like an incandescent light bulb, which emits essentially blackbody radiation. It is related to color temperature, in that the CRI measures for a pair of light sources can only be compared if they have the same color temperature. A standard "cool white" fluorescent lamp will have a CRI near 62."

The color temperature and CRI do not give the full picture. You also need to be aware of the radiation spectrum. Unfortunately, most gas discharge lamps have a spiked radiation spectrum that does not occur in nature. Due to this, you should avoid any artificial lighting that is created from gas discharge sources, such as mercury vapor, fluorescent, sodium, and so on.

Mercury based lighting mystifies me. We know that mercury is toxic to humans. So why would we make lighting products with it? In the future, mercury lighting products may be proven to be harmful to human health.

Stage lighting is known to affect some performers. Looking at bright stage lights for extended periods may eventually cause damage to the eye. This may eventually result in light sensitivity that is known as photophobia.

The next page shows how the florescent (mercury) and tungsten (traditional) light bulb spectrum's compare.

Florescent Spectrum

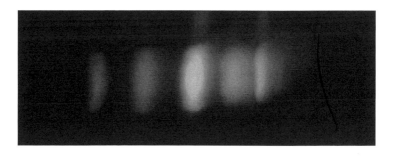

Note that the spectral lines are not continuous, but rather broken up. This is typical of gas discharge lighting. It does not occur in nature.

Tungsten Spectrum

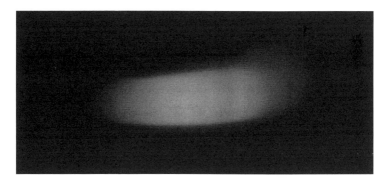

A smooth continuous spectrum that is typical of what nature produces.

Television, Computers & Phones

Televisions, computer displays and mobile phones are all sources of artificial light. You should be wary of your exposure to these as they may be able to impact your health.

The recent adoption of large screen televisions may bring with it an increase in human health problems in the future. People watching three dimensional images frequently may be an issue in the long term. Both of these could possibly be like a ticking time bomb. It is recommended that if you have a display in your environment that you keep it as small as possible. You may want to experiment with the brightness and contrast controls to get it to emit the lowest amount of light and still be comfortable to use. It is advised that your screen should not dominate your field of view.

Children who get addicted to video games have been documented as having the following problems:

- Depression
- Anxiety
- Social phobias
- Lower grades

The problems that displays can cause appears to be documented as computer vision syndrome (CVS). Computer vision syndrome (CVS) is a temporary condition resulting from focusing the eyes on a display for protracted, uninterrupted periods of time. People who wear glasses and contact lenses appear to have the highest frequency of this condition.

Some symptoms of CVS include:

- Headaches
- Blurred vision
- Neck pain
- Redness in the eyes
- Fatigue
- Disruption of the circadian cycle
- Eye strain
- Dry, irritated eyes
- Double vision
- Polyopia
- Difficulty refocusing the eyes.

Use your display in an environment that has good lighting in it and plenty of plants. Your display should not be the brightest thing in your environment.

Computers should have their screen designs to be largely a black background with white writing to enable the display to emit the lowest amount of radiation and to give high contrast. Computer anti-glare and security filters may be an issue also.

VR Displays & Microscopes

During the development of virtual reality (VR) displays it was noted that they were giving rise to severe vision problems and nausea. The newer eye-glass displays may produce vergence issues, where the eyes start to lose their ability to work together.

People who are working full time with microscopes are reporting problems with their health also. The National Board of Occupational Safety and Health in Sweden report, titled "Investigation of Visual Strain Experience by Microscope Operators at an Electronics Plant", concludes that 80% of microscope operators had visual strain. A statistically verified relationship was found to exist between visual eye strain and uncorrected astigmatism, poor eye coordination and time spent at the microscope.

Feeding the eyes with separate images and artificial light appears to cause problems and these effects may apply to three dimensional televisions in the future. Further study of these effects is desirable before three dimensional products become widespread.

New Lighting

I would recommend that you avoid the use of the new lighting that has been developed, such as gas discharge and light emitting diode (LED) lighting. These have been developed in order to use less energy at the expense of the quality of the light.

High intensity discharge (HID) lamps have appeared in projector televisions, public areas, warehouses, supermarkets, movie theaters, football stadiums, roads, parking lots and car headlamps. In cars, they have a blue appearance and have started to cause problems with other drivers due to their high intensity.

Ultra high performance high intensity discharge (UHP-HID) lamps that can be found in projector TV's may be a problem if they break as they contain mercury. This could be an issue in an enclosed space such as a house due to the mercury vapor that would be released into the air.

All artificial lighting should be generated by heat. This is how the Sun generates light. Unfortunately, there are no man-made sources of lighting that can generate the same temperature as the Sun. Halogen lighting is about as close as it gets and it is recommended that if you use artificial lighting that you use these types of lamps.

<u>Streetlights</u>

The streetlights that are present in modern society are polluting the view of the night sky and in most cities, it is barely visible. This may be a problem as it may interact with the eyes and the skin to cause unwanted effects in the body. It most likely will interfere with the circadian rhythm that governs the sleep cycle. Circadian problems are linked to:

- Depression
- Insomnia
- Cardiovascular disease
- Cancer

It is interesting to note that some diseases appear to be following the progress of electricity and night time lighting.

There are a number of definitions associated with nighttime lighting:

- Glare is created by light that shines horizontally
- Sky glow is the bright halo over cities at night
- Light trespass is light from one property spilling into another adjacent property

- Over-illumination is light that is far above what is needed for the activity

The International Dark Sky association can provide more details on this:

http://www.darksky.org/

Research on many types of wildlife shows that light pollution can alter behaviors, foraging areas and breeding cycles. The book "Ecological Consequences of Artificial Night Time Lighting" has more information on the subject.

Food Spoilage by Light

Supermarkets have known for a long time that light may cause food to spoil. In particular, supermarkets have realized that artificial lighting can accelerate the spoiling of the fresh food. The next time you are in the supermarket, take a look at the lighting in the fresh food section, it may well be different to that in the rest of the store. As such, they have identified lighting products that do not age the fresh food as quickly.

Spoilage of food by light is called photo-degeneration and it can cause problems with:

- Pigments
- Vitamin levels
- Fats
- Proteins

The density of the food will determine the depth of the photo-degeneration and liquids appear to be the most affected by it. Photo-degeneration can result in:

- Discoloration
- Off flavor
- Nutrient losses

Factors in photo-degeneration are:

- Light source strength
- Type of light
- Distance from the light source
- Length of exposure
- Optical properties of the packing materials
- Optical properties of the food
- Oxygen concentration of the food
- Temperature

The aging effect of light on food may have a similar effect in humans.

Colors & Moods

It has been known for a long time that colors can affect your mood. Now that the sunsets have turned orange and red, let us see what these colors produce in the human:

- Orange: Daring, stimulating
- Red: Stimulating, excitement, anger

It is recommended that you stay indoors during the time of the sunrise and sunsets. Watching the sky at this time may have health implications.

In locations that are nearer to the poles the Sun does not rise above the horizon very far. At these locations, there is a high level of atmospheric filtration taking place on the solar radiation during the daytime. Given the levels of pollution in the atmosphere, daytime may be bad for human health due to this level of filtration.

Good colors are :

- Yellow: Cheerful, positive
- Green: Calming
- Blue: Soothing
- Brown: Warm

Bad colors are:

- Red: Anger
- Violet: Rare in nature, regarded as artificial
- Black: Depressing, tired

Arranged in the color spectrum, we get:

- Infrared: Heat
- Red: Stimulating, excitement, anger
- Orange: Daring, stimulating
- Yellow: Positive
- Green: Calming
- Blue: Soothing
- Indigo: Deep contemplation
- Violet: Unnatural, rarely occurs
- Ultraviolet: Burns and damages skin

Looking at the color spectrum, we see that the center appears healthy while the outer limits appear unhealthy.

Full spectrum light is that which contains all of the colors as nature put them together. This is commonly referred to as white light. White is symbolic of purity and cleanliness. The opposite to this is black or no light.

Black is often associated with evil and death and is the color of fossil fuels.

Man-made lights that are used at night time are not full spectrum. As such, nighttime lighting or daytime office lighting should be kept as low as possible so that the human body does not absorb too much of it. In these environments it is advisable to use plants to modify the light to a natural form of light. The reflected light from plants may be essential to good human health.

Aggression

Humans have already started to figure out that nature is essential to good human health, as this United States Department of Agriculture article demonstrates:

Do Trees Strengthen Urban Communities, Reduce Domestic Violence?

By W. C. Sullivan, Ph.D. & Frances E. Kuo, Ph.D.

Cities are characterized by a whole host of social ills--from anonymity, to incivility, to outright violence--that are strikingly less prevalent in rural areas. Why is this? The physical environment a person lives in has profound effects on their social behavior. Social psychologists have shown that people in cities behave differently from people in rural areas in part because they live in crowded, noisy places, or in places that lack open space. But cities differ from rural areas in another important way as well--rural areas have something that's often lacking in urban areas--nature. Can part of the unsociableness of city dwellers be traced to the lack of plants in their everyday surroundings?

With support from the National Urban Community Forestry Advisory Council, we set out to answer these questions in one of the grimmest of urban settings--public housing in a major city.

As these pictures show, the number of trees immediately outside each of the 28 buildings at Robert Taylor Homes in Chicago vary considerably. Some buildings are surrounded only by concrete and asphalt, while others have trees, grass, and even flowers. Using aerial photographs and on-site analyses we chose 10 buildings with trees and 8 buildings without trees. We then interviewed 75 African-American women living in those buildings about their social behavior and compared the answers from women living in different buildings.

While the amount of plant life varies from building to building, very little else does. The buildings are architecturally identical. There are no systematic differences in the groups of people living in one building or another, perhaps because residents have very little choice in the specific apartment they are assigned. This gives us some confidence that differences we find in social behavior of people living in buildings with and without trees are really due to the trees--not differences in crowding, noise levels, or availability of open space, not differences in race, economic status, or even nature preferences in the people living there.

Do people who live in buildings with trees get along and treat each other better than people living in buildings without trees? The results of these interviews are not only interesting; they also provide new arguments in support of urban forest programs. Let's look at some of the highlights.

DO TREES STRENGTHEN URBAN COMMUNITIES?

For some time there have been stories about community gardens revitalizing inner city urban neighborhoods (Francis, Cashdan & Paxson 1984; Lewis 1972, 1979). Until now, however, no one has systematically examined the effect of trees on relations among neighbors.

We are finding signs of stronger communities where there are trees. In buildings with trees, people report significantly better relations with their neighbors. In buildings without trees, people report having fewer visitors and knowing fewer people in the building. In buildings with trees, people report a stronger feeling of unity and cohesion with their neighbors; they like where they are living more and they feel safer than residents who have few trees around them.

Why might trees contribute to better relations among neighbors? In 100 observations of outdoor common spaces in two public housing developments, we are finding that outdoor spaces with trees are used significantly more often than identical spaces without trees. We suspect that in urban areas, trees create outdoor spaces that attract people. When people are drawn to spaces with trees, they are more likely to see and interact with their neighbors, more likely to get to know each other and become friends.

Stronger ties among neighbors may be a good thing, but it becomes an even more convincing reason to support urban forests when you consider what neighborhood ties mean for residents' functioning. There is evidence that people with strong neighborhood ties are more physically healthy (Cassel 1976; Cobb 1976), more mentally healthy (Gottlieb 1983), less likely to neglect or abuse their children (Garbarino & Sherman 1980), and less likely to rely on costly social services in times of need (Biegel 1994; Gottlieb 1983; Collins & Pancoast 1976). In other words, these findings suggest that by investing in urban forests, a city might reap such dividends as a lowered incidence of child abuse, and decreased demand on social services.

DO TREES REDUCE VIOLENCE?

Two studies have shown a connection between trees and lower levels of violence (Mooney & Nicell 1992; Rice & Remy, in press). But these studies involved prison inmates, and Alzheimer patients living in nursing homes. What about people who are not living in institutional settings?

We are finding less violence in urban public housing where there are trees. Residents from buildings with trees report using more constructive, less violent ways of dealing with conflict in their homes. They report using reasoning more often in conflicts with their children, and they report significantly less use of severe violence. And in conflicts with their partners, they report less use of physical violence than do residents living in buildings without trees.

Why might trees contribute to less violence in the home? Imagine feeling irritated, impulsive, about ready to snap due to the difficulties of living in severe poverty. Having neighbors who you can call on for support means you have an alternative way of dealing with your frustrations other than striking out against someone. Places with nature and trees may provide settings in which relationships grow stronger and violence is reduced.

WHAT DOES THIS MEAN FOR URBAN FORESTRY?

In times of tight budgets, public officials look to reduce costs, and in doing so it is reasonable that they eliminate amenities. Trees have often been considered amenities. But what if urban foresters could report to city officials that trees help lower social service budgets, decrease police calls for domestic violence, strengthen urban communities, and decrease the incidence of child abuse in a city? Would the urban forest be considered an amenity then?

In this study, we are finding that urban forests help build stronger communities, and in doing so, they contribute to lower levels of domestic violence. Although no strong conclusions can be made from a single study, these findings are encouraging and exciting. At a time when the nation's attention is focused on issues such as crime prevention, health care, and the plight of single mothers, these findings suggest that trees can help address some of the most important problems in society today. We believe that urban forests are not mere amenities--that they are a basic part of the infrastructure of any city, as necessary as streets, sewers, and electricity.

REFERENCES

- Biegel, D.E. (1994). Help seeking and receiving in urban ethnic neighborhoods: strategies for empowerment. Prevention in Human Services. 3 (2-3): 119-143.

- Cassel, J. 1976. The contribution of the social environment to host resistance. American Journal of Epidemiology. 104(2): 107-123.

- Cobb, S. 1976. Social support as a moderator of life stress. Psychosomatic Medicine. 38(5): 300-314.

- Collins, A.H.; Pancoast, D.L. 1976. Natural helping networks: a strategy for prevention. Washington, DC: National Association of Social Workers.

- Francis, M.; Cashdan, L.; Paxson, L. 1984. Community open spaces: greening neighborhoods through community action and land conservation. Washington, DC: Island Press.

- Garbarino, J.; Sherman, D.1980. High-risk neighborhoods and high-risk families: the human ecology of child maltreatment. Child Development, 51(1): 188-198.

- Gottlieb, B.H. 1983. Social support as a focus for integrative research in psychology. American Psychologist. 38(3). 278-285.

- Lewis, C.A. 1972. Public housing gardens: landscapes for the soul. In Landscape for Living. Washington DC: United States Department of Agriculture Yearbook of Agriculture.

- Leuis, C.A. 1979. The sprouting of the inner city. Psychology Today. 13(1): 12-13.

- Mooney, P.; Nicell, P.L. 1992. The importance of exterior environment for Alzheimer residents: effective care and risk management. Gestion des soins de sante. Health Care Management forum: 5(2): 23-29.

- Rice, J.S.; Remy; L.L. (in press). Cultivating self development in urban jail inmates. Journal of Offender Rehabilitation.

Copies of this article and many others on human health and its relation to the trees can be obtained from the Landscape and Human Health Laboratory at the University of Illinois:

http://lhhl.illinois.edu/

Natural Light

So what functions are the trees performing that when they are not present will cause people to become aggressive?

The solar radiation interference effect that the tree canopy makes when solar radiation passes through it is probably the answer. This effect is called "Tree Canopy Light Interference". Light interference is a very big area of research in the optical and astronomical communities currently, it just has never been applied to the tree canopy.

Light is made up from waves and these waves can interfere with each other when passed through multiple apertures. The tree canopy makes many apertures that create the light interference effect. The result of this is that the solar radiation under the tree canopy is very different from the solar radiation above it. It is as different as night is to day.

Trees absorb the majority of the solar radiation and only reflect a small percentage of it back into the environment. They also change the color temperature and spectrum of the solar radiation. So to sum up, here are the effects that the tree canopy has on solar radiation:

- Interference of solar radiation

- Significant reduction in the power level of solar radiation
- Create a stable power level of solar radiation
- Color temperature modification of solar radiation
- Spectrum modification of solar radiation
- Conversion of solar radiation into natural energy
- Polarization of light

Without the tree canopy reducing and modifying the solar radiation, humans are subjected to flicker. This is an effect that is happening at sub-second speeds that is not noticed by the human eye. However, a high speed camera that shoots several frames per second can see this occurring. The Sun is basically increasing and decreasing its intensity due to atmospheric distortions and interference. Astronomers know this affect as "Astronomical Seeing". This effect may be able to induce dizziness, fatigue, headaches, epilepsy and nausea. Modern flicker may be a consequence of atmospheric pollution and may be far more severe than in the past.

An effect that is similar to this is broken clouds passing in front of the Sun. These produce extreme power cycles in the solar radiation levels The power levels can change by over 90% very quickly. The human body appears to have problems with this high level of frequent power cycling and again may experience dizziness, fatigue, headaches, epilepsy and nausea.

Solar radiation is made up of direct, diffuse and albedo radiation power levels. Direct is the view of the Suns disk, diffuse is the sky in general (the blue and/or cloudy part) and albedo is the reflections. Of these, direct contains over 90% of the energy and diffuse contains under 10%. There is no limit on the level that the reflections can be at and in a modern environment, such as a city, the albedo can increase the power levels many times of the sky based solar radiation of direct and diffuse combined.

Airy Disk Diffraction by Trees

The trees appear to produce the "Circle of Life" from diffraction and interference effects.

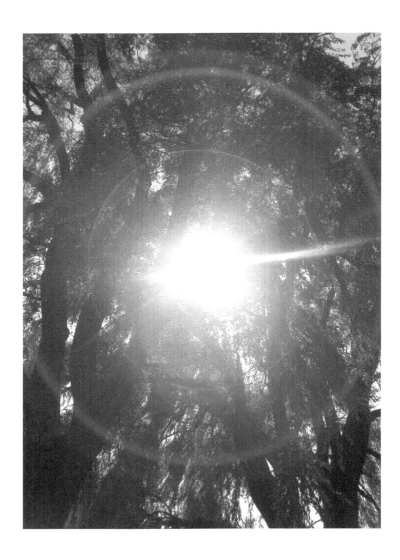

Lighting Levels

So what is a healthy level of lighting? If we take a look at the forest environment, then the answer is obvious. Keep lighting levels low and use plants in front of artificial lights to create light interference.

Over-illumination is a problem in the modern world and it may be able to affect your health. Keep it as low as possible and only increase lighting levels if you feel that you need more light in your environment. Use natural plants in front of your lights and windows to create light interference.

As for nighttime lighting, you should think candles! Not necessarily use candles, but rather the illumination level that candles create. There is a reason why candles are considered romantic and it is likely related to the low level of light that they create.

If you have your environment too bright during the nighttime, then you may upset the circadian rhythm that governs your sleep cycles. Keep lighting as low as possible during the nighttime. You should also keep your skin covered as much as possible to prevent it from absorbing the artificial light.

Incorrect radiation levels may be able to affect your sex drive and it may be proven in the future that human sex drive is governed more by radiation types and levels than any other factor, even more so than hormones!

Moonlight

Can moonlight affect your health? History says it can. The word "lunatic" is developed from the word "lune", which means Moon.

It appears that in the past, some people would go crazy if they were exposed to moonlight. This is documented as happening when someone would sleep in view of the Moon.

The Moon has a lighting level that is only 1/500,000 of the Sun. However, this reflected sunlight that the Moon creates is modified by the surface of the Moon and may be toxic to humans. There is a reason why the full Moon is associated with strange events!

The color temperature of the Moon is cooler than that of the Sun and therefore its light is very different from the Sun. The Moon emits a non-parallel form of light, also known as scattered light.

Vitamin D Deficiency

Sunscreens may block ultraviolet (UV) rays that produce vitamin D. There is growing concern that sunscreen may be harmful to human health. I currently advise people against the use of sunscreen. Rather, it is better to cover up and wear a wide brimmed hat. You do need some Sun exposure daily and I currently recommend that you spend as much time as you can in the shade of the trees for this exposure.

So why do they put vitamin D supplements in the food? Pollution can filter sunlight and may contribute to the development of rickets if you have insufficient dietary intake of vitamin D. You may, in some places, be getting poisoned by atmospheric pollution! The potential for this to occur is at its greatest in cities and industrial areas. To offset the pollution effect in humans, the vitamin D supplemented food is placed into the food supply.

Wikipedia states: In 1923, Harry Steenbock at the University of Wisconsin demonstrated that irradiation by ultraviolet light increased the vitamin D content of foods and other organic materials. After irradiating rodent food, Steenbock discovered the rodents were cured of rickets. A vitamin D deficiency is a known cause of rickets. Using $300 of his own money, Steenbock patented his invention. His irradiation technique was used for foodstuffs, most memorably for milk. By the expiration of his patent in 1945, rickets had been all but eliminated in the US.

Unfortunately, due to this filtering effect on sunlight, even spending time outside may not help you. You may need to take a trip of about 200 miles into the countryside to find healthy sunlight. It is a sad reflection on modern society that this was ever allowed to happen.

It is estimated that 36% of young people have vitamin D deficiency. 57% of hospital in-patients were found to be vitamin D deficient.

The medical conditions associated with vitamin D deficiency are:

- Rickets
- Osteomalacia
- Osteoporosis
- Diabetes
- High blood pressure
- Heart disease
- Colon cancer
- Various forms of cancer
- Multiple sclerosis

The symptoms of vitamin D deficiency include:

- Muscle weakness
- Legs may feel heavy
- Difficulty moving
- Aches and pains, may be severe
- Constant fatigue, even with sufficient sleep
- Moodiness
- Depression
- Anxiety
- Vomiting
- Nausea
- Diarrhea

If you have gone into the vitamin D deficient state, then you may notice that you get headaches that match changes in your solar radiation environment. This appears to be the body reacting to chemical changes that the sunlight exposure causes to it while it is in the deficient state.

People who live nearer to the poles generally have a higher chance of vitamin D deficiency. If you spend little time outdoors you may become vitamin D deficient. Unfortunately, modern society has increasingly become an indoor society which appears to be promoting the levels of vitamin D deficiency. If you have vitamin D deficiency, it is recommended to increase your daily outdoor time. By doing this you may cure your vitamin

D deficiency, as the human body can manufacture it from sunlight.

My research into low levels of solar radiation are indicating that it may cause high cholesterol, obesity and depression symptoms to occur in addition to low vitamin D. The links to low levels of radiation and other conditions may be extensive.

Solar Radiation Progression

This appears to be the current understanding of solar radiation power levels on the human body:

Too Low: Developmental problems, deformities in babies, bone deformity in the young, system deficiencies, low vitamin D, high cholesterol, hunger, obesity, anxiety, stress, mental issues, depression symptoms.

Normal: Unlimited energy during the day. Good sleep patterns. Excellent health.

High: Accelerated development, accelerated aging, going gray prematurely, hypochondriac symptoms, sleep problems, anxiety, stress, eye issues, mental issues, depression.

Too High: In addition to above: deformities in babies, bone deformity in the young (likely scoliosis), illness, onset of disease, most likely premature death.

Extreme: In addition to above: rapid onset of disease, major eye issues, premature death.

Unnatural sources of solar radiation (such as mercury lamps) may change the speed of progression of these problems and will most likely speed it up.

Constantly changing between the different levels (high cycling) may be able to induce mental instability or depression.

The definition of normal for humans is that of a forested environment in the tropics that has a tree canopy.

Human Eye

During the course of my research on solar radiation, I was also researching my own eyes. The conclusions that I came to are listed below.

- The eye is recessed to shelter it from the Sun
- The white (sclera) part of the eye is a bearing surface
- The colored area (iris) is for light absorption to prevent diffraction spikes
- The center (pupil) is a hole to allow light in
- The water cover (saline) of the eye has has these purposes:
  - Lubricate the bearing surface of the eye
  - Reflect excessive light
  - Act like a mirror to sunlight
  - Flush the eye when damaged
  - Keep the eye cool
  - Protect the structures of the eye from attack by bacteria and viruses
  - Act as a filter to solar radiation
- The eye has pain receptors that will activate when overloaded
- The overloaded eyes will start to flush

- The eyelids will involuntary close when the eyes are constantly overloaded
- The eyes will not be able to tolerate bright sunlight when constantly overloaded
- The only cure for constantly overloaded eyes is sleep and to stay in a dark environment until they recover, this generally takes a few days
- The eyes may not function perfectly for a few months after the overload as they progress towards a full recovery.
- Operating a computer may be difficult during the recovery period.

The human eye is coated in saline. Water is highly reflective when the Sun hits it at the correct angle. The human eye uses water to protect the eye from the Sun. The alignment of the human eye to the Sun will generally reflect sunlight from it.

Humans live in an environment where most of their time is spent looking either down or horizontal. The Sun is generally overhead when its power is strongest. As such, a wet eye surface will reflect much of the sunlight due to the angle that the sunlight would hit it at.

Water appears to have a cut-off filter effect that is angle dependent. The human eye seems to make use of this property.

If the human eye was dry, it would absorb far more of the sunlight and may be damaged by the Sun.

Constantly looking at the Sun will eventually overload the eye. To overload the eye in a short term direct view of the Sun appears to require the power of three Suns or a concentrated Sun.

The eyes connect directly into the brain through the optic nerves. The optic nerve may be incorrectly named, as it may actually be performing more functions than conventional nerves. It is possible that we may never fully understand how the eye, optic nerve and brain interact with each other.

The following pictures show the structure of the eye.

This is a photograph of the front of my eye. You will notice the reflection from the wet surface. The colored part (iris) of the eye absorbs and scatters light to produce a clear image through the center (pupil). The white part (sclera) of the eye is the bearing surface and is white to reflect light.

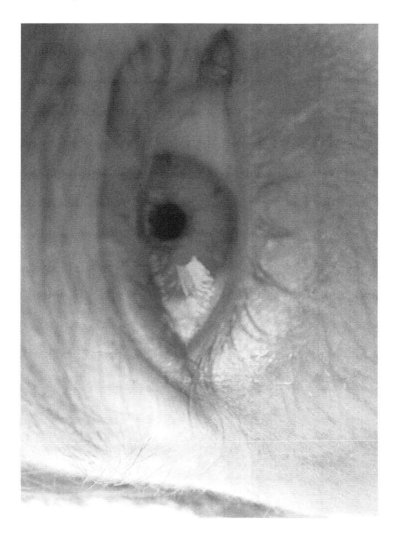

This is the side view of my eye. The eye is recessed to protect it from the Sun. The eyebrow and eye lashes absorb and scatter light that approaches the eye from outside of the field of view.

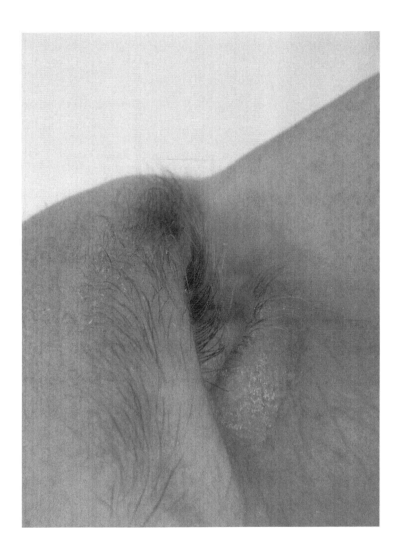

Human Eye Diagram

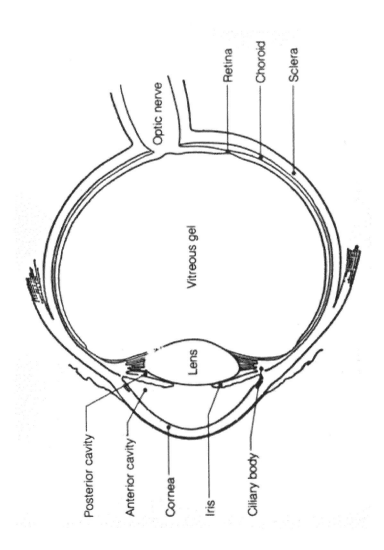

Eyes = Health Center

The eyes appear to be the health center of the human body. If the eyes are not receiving natural sunlight in the correct quantities daily, then the body may fall into illness and possibly progress onto a diseased state.

So what is the eye doing? It appears to have major functions in:

- Brain health
- Mental health
- Heart health
- General body health
- Sleep patterns
- Energy levels
- Cholesterol regulation
- Chemical composition of the blood
- Appetite

It is important that you do not filter the sunlight that the eyes receive when outdoors. Contact lenses, glasses and sun-glasses will filter light and should be removed when obtaining your daily outdoor exposure.

You should think of your eyes as solar modules that generate energy. Clearly, for them to generate positive energy, they need to be outdoors in the correct environment.

If your eyes do not receive the correct natural light, then you may become ill and eventually move into a diseased state. It is important that your eyes are fed the correct type of light and this appears to be the light that the forest canopy generates. This light is very different from a direct view of the Sun.

Low light and incorrect lighting environments appear to be able to cause low vitamin D, high cholesterol, obesity and fatigue. It appears that these conditions are linked together.

By feeding your eyes the incorrect types of light you may find that the brain function is affected, compromising your ability to think clearly and make effective decisions. In the future, I expect most forms of mental illness and depression to be proven to be linked to incorrect lighting environments.

It really should not be a surprise that the eyes and the brain interact so much, as they are almost the same thing, just the optic nerve separates them. I expect that in the future that the medical profession will recognize that when assessing mental health that the brain and the eyes must be considered together.

Night Vision

We may be born with the ability to see better in the night than what we currently can. Unfortunately, due to direct solar radiation in our society we may lose this nighttime light sensitivity during development.

It appears that our eyes were not made to function in an environment that has a direct view of the Sun. Rather, they were made to function in an environment where the solar radiation was modified by the trees and plants, and of a much lower power level.

Exposing our eyes to high levels of solar radiation will most likely damage them and we see evidence of this effect in the number of people who use contact lenses and glasses to correct their vision.

LASIK Eye Surgery

Laser-assisted in situ keratomileusis (LASIK) eye surgery is relatively new. It works by a machine cutting a flap in the cornea, lifting it up and then a laser re-figures the lens of the eye to the correct shape.

While it promises a restoration of normal eyesight, there are some problems with the technique. Some of these problems can be:

- Surgery induced dry eyes
- Overcorrection or under-correction
- Vitamin D deficiency from Sun sensitivity
- Visual acuity fluctuation
- Halos or starbursts around light sources at night
- Light sensitivity
- Ghost images or double vision
- Wrinkles in flap (striae)
- Decentered ablation
- Debris or growth under flap
- Thin or buttonhole flap
- Induced astigmatism
- Corneal Ectasia
- Floaters

- Epithelium erosion
- Posterior vitreous detachment
- Macular hole

The most common problem is dry eyes. The flap that is cut in the cornea generally will sever about 70% of the nerves to it. This affects tear production and lubrication of the eye. Six months after surgery about half of all patients are reporting problems with dry eye. Some patients never recover from the dry eye problems that LASIK can create. It is estimated that 40% of the nerves in the flap may never regenerate.

Some patients get a sensitivity to sunlight, called photophobia, and this may cause them to become vitamin D deficient due to avoidance of it.

Night time vision can be severely affected with star-bursts and halos in the field of view. This is a concern, as it means that diffraction and interference effects are taking place within the eye and this does not occur in a healthy eye. This appears to be caused by the scar tissue that forms after the surgery. Some patients are reporting that they cannot drive at night due to the interference effects in their night time vision.

A number of patients are reporting that their vision slips after a few years, sometimes becoming worse than the original problem. LASIK appears to suffer from aging effects in some cases.

Fatigue my be a problem in some patients and it is not clear if it is caused by the LASIK treatment.

Since LASIK is a relatively new technique that started to become popular in the 1990's, the long term effects of these problems has not fully emerged yet.

Blindness

When it comes to having the most knowledge about the human eye, the people who have it are actually blind! People who have had eye sight and then lost it are aware of the changes that it creates in the human body. These people fall into four categories:

- Blind in one eye
- Had one eye removed
- Blind in two eyes
- Have had both eyes removed

Blind people actually have the most problems with insomnia with eight out of ten blind people struggling to sleep.

The most common form of blindness is caused by vitamin A deficiency. It is rarely seen in developed countries but approximately 500,000 children go blind annually in less developed countries. About half of these die within a year of going blind. Vitamin A deficiency appears to be caused by not eating meat and night blindness is the first sign of the deficiency.

The most common forms of blindness are caused by:

- 47.8% Cateracts
- 12.3% Gloucoma
- 10.2% Uveitis
- 8.7% Age related macular degeneration (AMD)
- 5.1% Corneal opacity
- 4.8% Diabetic retinopathy
- 3.6% Trachoma

2.6% of the world's population are visually impaired. This subdivides into 2% have low vision and 0.6% are blind.

Diabetics have a high risk of eye problems, particularly cataracts and glaucoma. The most common threat to their vision is diabetic retinopathy.

Human Hair

Human hair protects the head from solar radiation. The head is the most exposed part of the body and it is important to keep it shaded from the Sun.

If you keep your hair short and you can see your scalp through it, then you will be receiving solar radiation through the skin in your scalp. If you are bald, then you perhaps may want to start wearing a hat to protect your head from solar radiation.

A large, wide brimmed hat is the best protection for both your head and your body from solar radiation. It creates shade wherever you go.

Be careful with your head, as it has the potential to receive the most solar radiation of any part of your body. Take appropriate precautions to keep yourself in good health and free of sunburn.

Human Skin

The human skin is referred to by many as the largest organ of the human body. As the largest organ, it also has the largest task in the body. It is your suit of armor against the environment and for it to work well requires attention on your part.

The human skin is sensitive to radiation. Expose it to solar radiation and it will start to react to it and make changes to the human body. The levels of radiation of all types needs to be controlled to natural levels in order for the changes that they create to be beneficial to humans.

The level of radiation that is recommended is that of the ground level vegetation environment under the tree canopy in the tropics. This is due to the "Tree Canopy Light Interference" effect.

The use of sunscreens are not recommended. There is much talk about sunscreen being potentially poisonous to the human body. Instead, use natural clothing such as white linen to keep the body covered and protected from solar radiation. It is interesting to note that human clothing styles changed significantly over the last century and prior to this it was normal to cover up the human body. Exposing lots of skin to the Sun is a relatively new trend in humans, as is sunbathing.

Many traditional cultures have understood the need to cover up the skin and, in men, to grow beards. Keeping hair to its natural length in all parts of the body appears to be a protector against radiation. Of interest is that hair may do this through the use of solar radiation interference as well as blocking the radiation.

You should keep skin contact of all man-made products to a minimum. Probably the only thing that should come into contact with your skin is natural clothing, natural materials (such as wood) and water. Avoid contact with plastics, metals, electronics, chemicals, soaps, make-up, and so on.

It is well known that the human skin protects us from solar radiation. It has several mechanisms that it uses in order to do this:

- Sweat is cooling
- Sweat is reflective
- Dried salt is reflective
- Skin changes color
- Different races will have different abilities to cope with high solar radiation environments

The medical profession has established that we need to expose our skin to solar radiation in order to produce essential vitamins. But exactly how much should you expose yourself to the Sun?

My current estimate is all day long in a natural rural environment with a tree canopy.

In a man-made environment, such as a city, I would not expose any skin to the direct view of the Sun. Rather you should use a wide brimmed hat and clothing to control your exposure to sunlight. This is due to the much higher solar radiation levels that are found in the cities. The city environment is extremely unpredictable and has areas of very high solar radiation.

In the future, cities may be signposted with signs that say: "Beware High Solar Radiation Area".

Human Health

Humans have been living on planet Earth for millions of years. The Sun has always been present and we are equipped to have long lives in its presence. For most of history we have led basic rural lives. In the last few hundred years that has changed with the migration of humans from the countryside into city living.

In the last two hundred years they have started to grow upwards into the sky. A global race started to claim the tallest building and with each decade, the buildings have grown further into the sky. Unfortunately, no one appeared to pay attention to the optical effects of these buildings and the human population in the streets below them.

Was this an unfortunate mistake in architecture? Around the world we now have buildings that have surfaces that are made of highly reflective glass and polished building materials. These buildings reflect extra sunlight into the human environment and it is currently unknown how this would affect human health in these cities.

At certain times of the day, modern cities have a sky view that contains multiple Suns. These multiple Suns do not seem to appear in nature and are now a concern for human health. Architects appear to have created an unnatural solar radiation environment in the world's cities.

This may cause an overload on the human body that may be similar to using drugs over an extended period. Toxins may build up in the body and it may not able to eliminate them due to continual frequent exposure to the higher than natural levels of solar radiation.

Wide brimmed hats and clothing can help keep the solar radiation exposure down on the human body.

Night time lighting is unnatural and may affect the human. It has been shown that away from night time lighting that the human sleep cycle changes. Two sleep cycles that are each about four hours long with a period of quiet rest appears to become the norm.

Over-illumination of both the daytime and nighttime environments is an issue to the human and also is an energy waste. One of the simplest ways of improving human health may be to reduce the lighting levels which also saves energy!

Unnatural radiation levels may cause problems in the human reproductive system. An interesting rumor in the airline industry is that pilots tend to father more females than males on average and this may be due to the radiation levels that they are exposed to. Infertility appears to becoming more of a problem and it may be linked to unnatural radiation levels.

Sunburn & Sunstroke

Sunburn is another name for solar radiation burn. There are two types of sunburn and these are natural and man-made.

Natural sunburn from the Sun is obtained in a natural environment free from man-made materials or development.

Man-made sunburn is a mix of natural reflections, man-made reflections, solar radiation diffraction and interference effects. These effects can be from buildings, cars, sidewalks, and so on. Man-made sunburn can also occur on tanning beds and from sun lamps and these should be avoided.

Man-made sunburn can be far stronger that natural sunburn and you need to be careful exposing yourself to sunlight in this environment. Sunburn can occur much quicker. The medical field has not documented this form of sunburn yet and until it does, you should exercise caution with sunbathing in these environments. Covering up is highly recommended.

All types of sun-burn may have long term effects that occur many years into the future.

When you sunbathe, you should keep a check on the environment that you are in. Many hotels reflect a lot of sunlight from their mirrored buildings onto the sunbathers below.

When exposing yourself to the Sun, you should check if you are taking any medications that may have reactions to sunlight. There are a surprising number of medications that will react to it.

When you get too much Sun, you may get the following medical conditions:

- Sunstroke presents with a hyperthermia of greater than 40.6°C (105.1°F) in combination with confusion and a lack of sweating. Symptoms can include dry skin, rapid, strong pulse and dizziness.
- Heat exhaustion can be a precursor of sunstroke. The symptoms include heavy sweating, rapid breathing and a fast, weak pulse.
- Heat cramps are muscle pains or spasms that happen during heavy exercise in hot weather.

Generally these occur in high solar radiation environments and can be a problem for outdoor workers. The solution is to move to a cool, low solar radiation environment and to rehydrate with electrolyte drinks. Prevention is better than cure and you should wear the correct clothing and be constantly hydrating when working outdoors.

Radiation Sickness

Radiation sickness occurs from high doses of radiation. This type of radiation sickness is well understood by the medical profession. However, there is a low level radiation sickness that is not well understood.

The effects of low level radiation exposure may cause random cancers, tumors and genetic defects many years into the future after exposure. No symptoms will initially be present during the exposure to the radiation source. It is like a silent killer.

Cancer and illness in our society appears to be random and can not currently be traced to a source.

Modern building techniques have increased the solar radiation levels in our society. This solar radiation peaks in cities with glass covered and mirrored buildings. These create powerful reflections from the Sun and increase the ground based solar radiation in the sidewalks and human environment. Sometimes there will be many different reflections of the Sun present from these modern buildings. This is called the "Multiple-Sun" effect.

The multiple-Sun effect does not appear to have been studied by the medical profession and the health implications are currently unknown.

Men Vs Women

It is surprising that in the United Kingdom women have greater levels of cancer than men in almost all areas of the human body. This may be due to women exposing more of their skin due to current society fashion trends. Women tend to wear low cut tops and short skirts.

Women can generally be found to be sunbathing more than men in an effort to improve their appearance.

These habits that women have formed with exposing more skin appear to cause greater radiation absorption for the female body.

Indeed, breast cancer is at extremely low levels in men when compared to women. Women typically display their breast skin to the environment due to fashion and cultural trends. Men generally do not. The much higher levels of radiation exposure that women receive to the breasts may be a cause for the increased cancer rate. Breast cancer is the top cancer in women in the United Kingdom.

The breasts on most female animals face the ground and are shielded from the Sun due to the use of four legs in the animal world. Exposing the breasts to direct solar radiation may be an unnatural habit that is unique to humans.

Humans are relatively hairless animals. It is this lack of hair that allows humans to receive a lot of solar radiation when compared to the majority of land based animals. We have developed clothing to replace this lack of hair on our bodies. It is important that we mimic animals and use our clothing to cover our skin from direct sunlight. This can be done by wearing layers of clothing to ensure that the solar radiation that penetrates the clothing and reaches the skin is of a low power level.

Males and females probably have different abilities to cope with solar radiation due to the differences in hormones.

Women appear to suffer more from headaches than men. This may be due to having more skin exposed to solar radiation and therefore more absorption of it. Women appear to be more aggressive than in the past and this may contribute to it.

Pain

The sixth human sense is that of pain. It is the alarm system of the human body. To ignore it is like committing suicide. You will only get worse, not better. Humans have invented the pharmaceutical industry to override this system of pain so that humans can keep working, instead of recovering at home. Do not ignore pain!

Most people get general aches and pains. These people had been labeled as hypochondriacs by the medical profession. We now know that the medical profession may be wrong and that most people with general aches and pains are perhaps suffering from the effects of poisoning, most likely radiation poisoning.

Do not ignore your pains, they are very real. You need to take action and locate the source of the problem in your environment and remove it to return to good health. A prescription to override it will most likely send you to an early grave. There is a saying in the medical profession "Inside every tablet is a little bit of poison". Avoid medications if you can.

<u>Aging</u>

Solar radiation is an oxidant and can cause aging. Indeed the Center for Disease Control (CDC) already has solar radiation listed as a carcinogen.

The aging effects of solar radiation may include:

- In children it may cause accelerated development into puberty
- In women it may be able to accelerate the onset of menopause
- Hair may go gray prematurely
- Dry hair
- Wrinkles may start to appear
- Skin structure may start to change
- Hair may start to thin
- Accelerated aging
- Eyes may prematurely fail
- Tooth decay

If you notice that your body appears to be aging prematurely, you would be wise to survey the environments that you pass through during a typical year and assess the levels of radiation that are present in them.

Unnatural radiation environments that are identified should be either avoided or passed through quickly. Good selection of clothing and hats can help to reduce exposure to unnatural levels of radiation.

Depression

Depression may appear in the human body if large changes in solar radiation exposure occur. This is currently documented in the medical field as seasonal affect disorder (SAD). People may go into depression as the sunlight exposure levels reduce as the seasons transition from summertime to wintertime. It is common for doctors to prescribe light treatments for people who experience this.

The human body appears to pass through a depression period and into good health in about two months and this will vary on the individual. Returning from a low sunlight exposure level back to a high sunlight exposure level may trigger a depression effect again.

This may be diagnosed in people who vacation to different climates. The solar radiation change appears to cause illness initially until the body adjusts to the different level. This apparent illness is commonly reported as tiredness, colds, headaches, insomnia, food poisoning or a change in the drinking water quality.

It may be possible to control and perhaps prevent certain human depression disorders by keeping sunlight exposure levels low and relatively constant throughout the year. It is far easier to maintain a low level solar radiation environment than a high level environment. It is also healthier to be in the low level environment for skin cancer prevention.

Obesity may result when in a depressed state due to over eating and a lack of exercise. Depression appears to be the body's way of reacting to change. If you are constantly exposing your body to change then it may stay in a depressed state continually.

The hunger effect that is observed in humans that leads to obesity appears to be due to an imbalance in chemical composition in the human body. When a chemical imbalance is present, the human body triggers hunger in order to try and extract the needed chemicals from the food that you eat. Unfortunately, if it cannot rectify the chemical imbalance, then the desire to eat will not subside. This will lead to obesity.

Feeding your body the correct light nourishment appears to eliminate the hunger effect. The light that appears to suppress hunger is that generated by the tree canopy.

Mental Illness

Mental illness is defined as any of various disorders in which a person's thoughts, emotions, or behavior are so abnormal as to cause suffering to himself, herself, or other people

Solar radiation, modified solar radiation and artificial radiation may be able to cause mental illness. The combination of these is unnatural and may explain the increasing number of mental illness cases that we see in society today. The UK reports that in the last four years alone (2006-2010), prescriptions for mental health drugs have gone up 40%!

Why would this be? When you measure the solar radiation under the tree canopy you find that it has a very low power level of about 100 watts per square meter. If you step out from under the tree canopy and measure the direct view of the Sun, it will have a power level of about 1,130 watts per square meter at solar noon in the tropics at summertime. This is approximately eleven times more energy that you are subjecting your body too. The radiation types are also very different, as the tree canopy creates interference solar radiation.

The level of solar radiation that can be found in cities can exceed that of Space. If you are in an environment that has extremely high levels of solar radiation, then you should not be surprised if you fall into ill health. While the health effects of extremely high solar radiation are currently unproven, it is extremely high levels of energy that you may be exposing yourself to in this environment.

Technology is becoming more prevalent in the office, car and home environments and the technologies in the displays keeps changing. They are increasing their physical screen sizes, contrast ratios, resolutions, pixel size and brightness. This may be one of the reasons for the increasing rates of mental illness.

Gulf War Syndrome

Gulf war syndrome is being reported by troops who are returning from tours of duty in the desert regions. No one really understands why they are getting ill. They typically report the following problems:

- Heart problems
- Severe pains in muscles and joints
- Chronic fatigue
- Headaches
- Sleep disturbances
- Irritable bowl
- Stomach issues
- Respiratory issues
- Psychological problems

The desert regions generally have the some of the highest solar radiation levels in the world. Some factors that may apply to this condition are:

- The soldiers genetics are generally incompatible with the solar radiation in the region
- Solar radiation interference effects from turbulence in the atmosphere that is caused by the high temperature levels

- Solar radiation interference effects from dust storms
- The use of high factor sunscreens

It is plausible that toxic light may be contributing to Gulf War Syndrome.

Withdrawal Symptoms

When the body is changing from a high solar radiation exposure to a low solar radiation exposure quickly, the following symptoms may be present:

- Perception of hot skin pains that are similar to sunburn
- Insomnia
- Chest pains
- Intestinal pains
- Head pains
- Pains may be severe
- Headaches, may last several days
- Random sensory nerve pains
- Random motor nerve twitches
- Changes in stools
- Cold symptoms

It is recommended that if you choose to move into low solar radiation exposure, that this be done gradually over the period of one year and under the supervision of a licensed and qualified medical physician.

This can be done by wearing a wide brimmed hat and slowly increasing opaque clothing levels. If it is done too quickly, the body may experience a depression reaction with non-specific general pains.

Once in the low level it is recommended to keep it there. You should try and stay in a natural shaded environment of tree cover when outside.

If it moves from low to high (not recommended) the following problems may occur:

- Tiredness
- Insomnia
- Stress
- Headaches
- Upset stomach
- Diarrhea
- Intestinal pains
- Joint pains
- General pains
- Depression
- Cold symptoms
- Hyperactivity
- A state of mind similar to intoxication at times

Radiation Poisoning

Radiation poisoning may have many stages to it, each with its own set of conditions. It may use obesity to build up a layer of fat in order to protect the nerves, internal organs, muscles, circulatory system and skeleton from radiation damage.

It is important to keep an open mind until more is known by the medical profession. Until proven otherwise, any disease or disorder in human society may have a link to radiation poisoning.

Brain disease appears to be on the increase in humans and it may be linked to unnatural levels of radiation in the human environment.

The indoor environment that most modern humans have adopted may actually be harming them. The human appears to be an outdoor forest animal by genetics and therefore being indoors during the daytime appears to be an unnatural activity. In the absence of natural solar radiation, the body appears to try to absorb radiation from the indoor environment and this may make humans ill. This creates the possibility of radiation poisoning to occur.

High Risk Humans?

Who is at greatest risk? People exposed to a direct view of the Sun's broad spectrum radiation include:

- Agricultural workers

- Farmers

- Horticultural workers

- Maintenance workers

- Pipeline workers

- Ranchers

- Athletes

- Fishermen

- Landscapers

- Painters

- Window cleaners

- Military personnel

- Police

- Ski instructors

- Brick masons

- Gardeners

- Lifeguards
- Oilfield workers
- Postal carriers
- Sailors
- Construction workers
- Greens-keepers
- Loggers
- Open-pit miners
- Railroad track workers
- Surveyors
- Roofers
- Green jobs
- Pilots
- Drivers
- Car park attendants
- Auto sales people
- Cyclists
- Electrical line workers
- Electrical switch yard workers
- Communication line workers

- People who spend time next to a window
- People who have large amounts of skin exposed
- People who wear thin clothing that is relatively transparent to solar radiation
- Anyone who regularly passes through areas of high levels of solar radiation
- People who walk the dog regularly
- People who live in houses that generate high levels of man-made solar radiation
- High altitude workers
- High altitude living
- Anyone who does not have vegetation in their environments

People who are exposed to high levels of artificial radiation are:

- Hospital workers
- Office workers
- Night shift workers
- Submariners
- Restaurant workers
- Shop workers
- Warehouse workers

- Miners
- Computer operators
- Stage performers
- Radio transmission engineers

Healthy Habits

Reasonable precautions are:

- Keep solar radiation exposure natural
- Avoid eye wear of any type when obtaining your outdoor daily solar radiation exposure.
- Avoid sunlamps and tanning beds
- Wear UV sun-glasses in unnaturally high solar radiation environments
- Use sunscreen on exposed parts of the body during daytime in unnaturally high solar radiation environments
- Do not wear make-up
- Wear a wide brimmed hat
- Use an umbrella to create shade
- Seek shade
- Cover up your body with layers of opaque clothing
- Wear collared, long sleeve shirts to provide arm and neck coverage
- Learn to recognize high albedo locations
- Learn to look for the multiple-Sun effect
- Take note of locations that should be avoided due to high solar radiation levels

- Avoid open spaces
- Avoid driving into sunrises and sunsets
- Eat fresh fruit and vegetables often
- Avoid medications and vitamin supplements
- Control your solar radiation environment to prevent large changes in solar radiation levels received by your body
- Drink filtered tap water

Above all, don't panic. People have been living in cities for years and many live long lives.

You should obtain your daily solar radiation exposure during the peak hours which are generally regarded as an hour after sunrise through to an hour before sunset.

You must remember that both sunglasses and sunscreen are predominantly filtering the UV radiation component of sunlight. They do not offer full protection against the content of broad spectrum solar radiation. This filtered solar radiation may not be healthy for the human body.

You can do a light test on your clothing by holding it up to the Sun and seeing how much sunlight passes through it. You may be quite surprised at how transparent you clothing actually is! You should identify the transparency of your clothing and use layers of it in order to reduce the transparency. Some transparency is desirable to enable skin absorption of solar radiation. Thin clothing should be worn in low solar radiation environments and denser clothing should be worn in high solar radiation environments.

In the future, clothing should be labeled as to how it blocks the full solar radiation spectrum, similar to how sunscreen and sunglasses are labeled today. Most clothing will not prevent the entire broad spectrum solar radiation from reaching the skin.

People with long hair have an advantage as the body has hair for solar radiation protection. Wearing your hair long will help protect you from solar radiation effects. Cutting hair is a relatively modern phenomenon and if left uncut it will generally grow to the full length of the back. It appears to be important for humans to protect the back from solar radiation and this is probably due to the spinal cord being in this location. Most animals appear to have fur (hair) and this may be for solar radiation protection.

You should assess the solar radiation environments where you pass through during a typical year. You should make adjustments accordingly to any areas of high solar radiation levels to bring them down to a normal level. If you are unable to bring solar radiation levels down in some areas, then these areas should either be avoided or appropriate protection should be worn in these areas.

Reverse Aging

When you start following the guidelines you may notice reverse aging taking place. This may be due to the stresses being reduced from the human body and it returning to a more natural level of solar radiation absorption.

In modern society, there are many people who have incorrect solar radiation exposure. The indoor office environments of modern society with their florescent lights and personal computer systems are one of the more toxic light environments that you can place your body into.

It is important that if you are in one of these toxic light environments that you do obtain natural sunlight exposure and it is recommended that you do so daily in the nearest environment that has trees that create shade.

Human Environment

We have established that the majority of humans are living in the incorrect environments. So what is the correct environment?

Historians indicate that the humans started out in the tropics in Africa. The tropics in Africa is a lush forested environment with a tree canopy. The tropics has a stable year round climate. They were under the tree canopy, as they would have have been burned by the Sun without clothes in the open.

Science has proven that the trees and plants reduce and modify the radiation levels to make them healthy to humans. Eating the fruits and vegetables is known to prevent free radicals from occurring inside the human body and keeps the body young.

At this point we have our answer. The human environment is supposed to have the following characteristics:

- Tropical
- Tree canopy
- Tree interference solar radiation
- Low solar radiation levels

- Lots of vegetation
- Stable, year round, warm temperatures
- A source of natural surface water
- A source of natural food

This can be summed up by concluding that the human may have the genetics of a forest animal.

To move away from this type of environment is likely to induce pain, illness and disease into the human body. This has been demonstrated by the high amounts of it in modern society. Environments that are devoid of green spaces are associated with greater levels of childhood obesity, higher rates of disease, and higher rates of mortality in young and the elderly.

Greener environments have been shown to aid recovery from surgery, enable and support higher levels of physical activity, improve immune system functioning, help diabetics achieve higher blood glucose levels, and improve functional health status and independent living skills amongst older adults.

The human body develops in the environment where the person was raised. If the person significantly changes that environment, then it may raise the risk of illness.

Humans can be found in every climate zone on the Earth. They are the only animal that has complete climate zone coverage. The rest of the animals stay within their genetic climate zones, as they know they will get ill outside of them.

Could you imagine a polar bear at the Equator or a pink flamingo at the North Pole? They would surely die in these locations. It's strange that humans cannot see this effect in their own species.

Correct Radiation Levels?

So what are the correct solar radiation levels for a human? This is something that is based on the individual, their genetics and their global location. It is unique to each person and you will only be able to establish your correct level by experimentation.

A common number that you hear is fifteen minutes per day. This appears to be incorrect, as the human appears to be an outdoor forest animal by genetics. I was able to produce symptoms of extreme tiredness with just a fifteen minute daily exposure, which confirmed that the outdoor exposure time is much higher.

Here are some estimates that I developed in Tucson, Arizona, USA and they are for guidance only:

- Forest environment with a dense tree canopy:
  - All day exposure under the tree canopy.
- Green rural environment without a tree canopy:
  - Four hours in the shade of the nearest trees.
- City environment:
  - You should avoid solar radiation exposure in a city due to the large number of reflections, diffraction and interference effects that may be present. You should wear a wide brimmed hat

in this environment. If you need to get sunlight exposure in a city location then you should obtain your exposure in the park in the shade of the trees.

These numbers were developed by obtaining exposure while wearing a long sleeve shirt and trousers. My head was exposed, I had a short beard and my hands were not covered.

If you don't get sufficient daily outdoor solar radiation exposure, then you may move into a unnatural and possibly depressed state. You will know when you are in a really low a state of radiation exposure as you will start to get frequent headaches that match your changing radiation levels. If you are getting frequent headaches, then it is recommended that you increase your outdoor exposure to sunlight to bring it back up to normal levels.

It is important that when you obtain your outdoor exposure that you wear a wide brimmed hat when in the direct view of the sun, due to the high power of it. You should not wear makeup, sunscreen nor any type of eye wear. This includes contact lenses, glasses and sunglasses. To prevent yourself from burning you should use white natural clothing when in a direct view of the sun. Both hands and face should be exposed to the environment.

The problem with the direct view of the Sun is that the power level is too high for the human body. This shows up as sunburn and possibly sunstroke. You should create your own shade in this environment by using a wide brimmed hat and white clothing. White clothing will keep you cool as it reflects the radiation. I do not recommend sunscreen as it will filter the radiation and creates an artificial form of radiation that may be harmful to the human body.

There is a simple test that you should use daily. In the evening you should take a look at your skin and see if there is sunburn anywhere. If there is, then you passed through an environment that the radiation levels were too high for your body. You should identify the environment and take the appropriate precautions next time.

Given the modern culture that we live in, it is easy to find yourself in the depressed state of incorrect solar radiation exposure. This may occur if you do not spend sufficient time outdoors.

The following are not outdoor exposures:

- Driving a car, truck, or tractor
- Sitting indoors next to a closed window
- Artificial lighting
- Sunbeds or tanning lamps

You should keep track of true outdoor exposure and make sure that whatever environment that you are in, that you are getting sufficient outdoor time to keep yourself in good health. You should increase the outdoor time based on weather conditions such as clouds.

You should be wary of artificial lighting as your body will absorb it. There is no artificial lighting that is equivalent to the Sun. In the future, some types of artificial lighting may be proven to be able to affect human health.

The same is true of glass. All glass acts like a filter to solar radiation. In the future certain types of glass may be proven to be harmful to human health.

Displays of all types produce artificial radiation. You should count the hours per day that you are exposed to these and you should aim to keep it to a minimum. Watching television or operating a computer should not become a regular habit.

Artificial radiation exposure may lead to random pains, depression symptoms and possibly onto disease. You should avoid artificial radiation exposure.

Children

Children should be protected from direct Sun. Here are some suggestions to effectively do this:

- Bedrooms should face the Pole, no direct solar radiation should come into the room
- Playrooms should face the Pole, no direct solar radiation should come into the room
- Outside play areas should be shaded by native trees and face the pole
- Clothing should cover up as much skin as possible and should be layered
- Children should wear a large, wide brimmed hat when outdoors
- Children should be shaded when outdoors
- Glass and reflective surfaces should be covered
- They should not use sunscreen when obtaining their daily solar radiation.
- They should not wear any type of eye wear when obtaining their daily solar radiation.

Things to watch for in children:

- Hyperactivity

- Depression
- Learning difficulties
- Lack of friends and social contact
- Aggression
- Development problems
- Illness
- Weird behaviors
- Cold symptoms
- Upset stomach
- Diarrhea
- Intestinal pains
- Colic
- Accelerated development into puberty
- Eye problems

If you see any of these, it may be that your child has changed levels of solar radiation exposure and absorption. The recommended solution is to place them into a known healthy solar radiation environment. I currently recommend under the tree canopy in the forest. The solar radiation environment is to be kept as constant as possible during the daytime. Avoid large swings in daily solar radiation levels.

Feng Shui

Feng Shui is the study of positive energy in the human environment. It literally means wind and water. The people who developed Feng Shui understood that human emotions and health were governed by their environments. Good lighting and quality air are the basics of Feng Shui.

Mal-illumination was a term used by John Nash Ott to describe sunlight deficiency and the harmful effects of florescent lighting on human health, behavior and learning abilities. He is quoted as saying "Light is to mal-illumination as food is to malnutrition.".

Your body reacts to the energy around you and it either nourishes you or drains you. If you are feeling ill or having emotional issues, you should apply the science of Feng Shui to your environment as it will probably help a lot. Light is regarded as the medicine of the future.

You can't go wrong by having an environment that has the science of Feng Shui applied to it. This environment should be a natural green environment of plants and trees with natural sunlight. We see this in children who are instinctively drawn to green environments. Simply opening the windows in your house and letting natural light and air into it may be able to improve your health.

John Nash Ott

John Nash Ott became well known for his time-lapse photography of plants that were featured in a number of Walt Disney productions. He pioneered the technique and became well known for his amazing films of plants growing from seeds to full size in just a few minutes. The "Secrets of Life" (1956) film series featured his work.

John Nash Ott extensively studied plants and how they interact with light, indeed he was one of the pioneers in the field of photo-biology. His experiments showed that plants would not grow well under artificial lights unless they were full spectrum lighting products. Plants grown under other forms of light would show stress. In particular, he found that plants grown under all common florescent tubes would mutate and form unnaturally.

He found that he could manipulate the growth of plants by varying the color temperature of the light to cause:

- Flowering
- Fruiting
- Changing gender

He progressed onto experimenting with animals and individual cells, and he realized that the same effects would likely occur in humans. Stress would occur without natural outdoor sunlight in living organisms that included humans. He concluded that all life needed the full spectrum of outdoor sunlight to thrive. This included the ultraviolet and infrared parts of the spectrum.

He discovered that the color temperature of light could affect human mental heath and that full spectrum lighting reduced hyperactivity in the classroom and also negative behavior in prison and mental health facilities. He realized that the light that enters the eyes has a function in regulating the brain chemistry and will affect how we feel and function.

His research indicated that there may be dangers in the overuse and under-regulation of modern electromagnetic technology. Of interest is that he found problems with:

- Digital watches
- Certain man made fibers such as polyester and vinyl
- Ionizing-type smoke detectors
- Certain types of fluorescent lighting
- Video display terminals
- Electronic fetal monitoring equipment in hospitals
- Other high technology items
- Relationship of colored lighting and the positive and negative effects that it can create.

In the 1980's, he published a series of seven articles in the International Journal of Bio-social Research under the title of "Color and Light: Their Effects on Plants, Animals, and People". In these articles he promoted the benefits of obtaining full spectrum sunlight in an outdoor environment.

My research into solar radiation and human health is matching that of John Nash Ott and it was performed independently of his research. I only became aware of his extensive research into the area during proof reading Toxic Light and added this chapter just before I copyrighted the book.

His books have more information on the subject of health and sunlight:

- My ivory cellar; [the story of time-lapse photography] (1958)
- Health and Light: The Extraordinary Study That Shows How Light Affects Your Health and Emotional Well Being. (1973)
- Light, Radiation, and You: How to Stay Healthy (1982)
- Color and Light: Their Effects on Plants, Animals and People (1985)

He has also produced a movie on the subject:

- Exploring the Spectrum: The Effects of Natural and Artificial Light on Living Organisms (1960's)

Astronomy

Astronomy is the study of the universe, including our solar system. Most professional astronomers study the stars. The Sun and the Moon have largely been ignored by the astronomical communities for a number of decades now. This appeared to coincide with the ending of the NASA Moon mission program.

Astronomers have moved the majority of their facilities above the pollution, filtering and turbulence effects of the atmosphere. Astronomy facilities are now commonly found on mountain tops with elevations of seven thousand feet through to about fifteen thousand feet.

The result of this is that most astronomers disconnected from the effects of atmospheric pollution and ground based radiation levels, as they were no longer really affected by it. The ignorance that astronomers have displayed with ground based radiation in the human environment will be regarded as the biggest mistake ever made in the astronomical community.

Astrology

Astrology is the study of our solar system as it relates to human emotions. Its premise is that human emotions are related to the movements of the solar system. Human emotions are definitely affected by the Sun and probably also by the Moon. The Planets also appear to have an effect. In the absence of street lights, it is probable that starlight would interact also.

Most humans will recognize astrology as the horoscopes that are displayed in the newspapers and magazines. They appear to indicate things that will happen in your life that are related to your birth sign. It is likely that given the amount of light pollution that is present in today's societies that astrology predictions may not be as accurate as they were in the past.

When you work in the professional astronomy community, you realize that there is an absence of astrologers. It appears that astronomers and astrologers don't mix and have developed separate fields of study. This has been a mistake and should be rectified. Astronomy and astrology are completely related subjects and one cannot be taught without the other.

Research into solar radiation in the human environment is indicating a strong link between human emotions and the Sun.

Summary

The human appears to be an outdoor forest animal by genetics that has decided to be an indoor animal. Unfortunately, this does not appear to match its genetics and the indoor society appears to be making people ill in large numbers.

As individuals, we can control our own natural environments. Our houses should be under the tree canopy. Windows should have plants next to them on both the inside and outside. The gardens of our homes should be like forests. The inside of our homes should be filled with plants. The outside of our homes should be dark, non-reflective natural colors. Our work environments should be filled with plants and natural lighting. The top thing that you can do to stay in good health or improve your health is to surround yourself with plant life and natural sunlight. This includes eating live plant foods such as salads, raw vegetables and fruits.

A natural green environment has been shown to improve mental health, increase self discipline and impulse control. Less access to nature is related to increased attention deficit and hyperactivity disorder symptoms, higher rates of anxiety disorders, and higher rates of clinical depression.

Direct beam solar radiation, a direct view of the Sun, contains over ninety percent of the solar radiation energy that is received at ground level. We must block this direct view with trees that convert the energy naturally. This will result in a cooler ground level environment that is conducive to good health in humans with the best light nutrient.

Trees are solar radiation absorbers and suppressors and we must start replanting native trees, especially so in the human environments. The schools would be a good place to start so that the solar radiation levels around the young are reduced back to natural levels. Reducing the solar radiation levels may allow the human body to repair any damage that may have occurred from exposures to high levels of it.

Humanity needs to be in the presence of a tree canopy in order to be a peaceful race. The trees appear to prevent us from developing illness and disease, the trees have a lot of power over us. As such, we need to spend time evaluating the relationship of the natural environment to that of a modern man-made environment.

Climate change is very real and has the potential to lead to human extinction. It is now reasonable to state that climate change has progressed into Earth change. The Earth appears to be entering a period of unrest that has not been observed in recent centuries.

As individuals, we can control the direction of the human race. It is recommended that you ensure that the leaders of the nations have the natural world and human health at the top of their agenda's. Use your vote wisely, your childrens future is at stake. We are the masters of our childrens future. It is recommended that the children voice their desires for the future to their parents.

Be healthy by being outdoors in the sunlight with nature!

This book is not a substitute for professional medical advice from a qualified and licensed medical physician. You should always consult a professional when making lifestyle changes or if you suspect that you have an illness.

Definitions

Sunlight

- Sun: Our closest star, a giant nuclear reactor in the sky.
- Natural Sunburn: Sunburn from the Sun and reflections from nature.
- Man-Made Sunburn: Sunburn from the Sun and a mix of natural and man-made reflections and optical effects.
- Full Spectrum: Sunlight that contains the full ultraviolet, optical and infrared spectrum as it occurs in nature.
- Direct: Sunlight that occurs in the sky where the view of the Suns disk is.
- Diffuse: Sunlight that occurs across the rest of the sky, excluding the Suns disk.
- Albedo: Sunlight that occurs from reflections from ground based objects.

Multiple-Sun Effect

- Multiple-Sun: Two or more Suns are present.
- Stereo-Sun: Two Suns are present that are opposite each other.

- Surround-Sun: Three or more Suns are present around you.
- Light-maze: A grouping of glass covered buildings that sunlight bounces around in.
- Lighthouse: A reflected Sun that follows you as you move around the building.

Light

- Parallel Light: Light that travels in parallel.
- Semi-Parallel Light: Light that travels in a similar direction with some scattering present.
- Non-Parallel Light: Scattered light with no bright areas.
- Filtered Light: Light that has reduced its power level and may have lost parts of the full spectrum.
- Reflected Light: Light that has been reflected from a surface and has taken on the spectral properties of that surface.
- Polarized Light: A type of light that can occur by filtration or reflection which causes polarity.
- Chromatic Aberration: Occurs when light passes through a medium and starts to exhibit fringes of color.
- Diffraction: Occurs when parallel light passes over an object which causes the light waves to start spreading outwards.

- Interference: Occurs when spreading light waves start to cross with each other and interact.
- Glare: Created by light that shines horizontally.

Streetlights

- Sky Glow: The bright halo over cities at night.
- Light Trespass: Light from one property spilling into another adjacent property.
- Over-Illumination: Light that is far above what is needed for the activity.

References

- Do Trees Strengthen Urban Communities, Reduce Domestic Violence? Paper by By W. C. Sullivan, Ph.D. & Frances E. Kuo, Ph.D.
- Google Maps http://maps.google.com/
- Investigation of Visual Strain Experience by Microscope Operators at an Electronics Plant. Paper by Occupational Safety and Health, Sweden
- John Nash Ott http://www.biolightgroup.com/Ott.html
- National Renewable Energy Laboratories www.nrel.gov
- Wikipedia http://www.wikipedia.org/

Acknowledgements

This book was influenced by a caring person that I wish to thank:

- Claudia Sandoval for her wisdom on trees and how it relates in the social environment.

About the Author

Steven started his career at one of the largest university research hospitals in Europe. Working in the electrical engineering group, he obtained a Bachelors with Honors in Electrical and Electronic Engineering. Human health was a strong draw and he moved into the biomedical team, serving the regions hospitals. During this time he developed a fascination for human disease and the causes of it, many of which were not understood.

He joined the Isaac Newton Group of Telescopes in 1999 and went to live in La Palma. La Palma is part of the Canary Islands, governed by Spain. During this time he worked with the leading European astronomers and developed his astronomical and optics skills. He became fluent in Spanish and their culture.

In 2001 he joined the W. M. Keck Telescopes in Hawaii. This was the world's leading astronomical facility and home to the world's two largest segmented mirror telescopes. Steven developed segmented optics and interferometry skills while working alongside world leading astronomers. During this time Steven constructed his own off-grid solar powered home in the last of the traditional Hawaiian fishing villages in Miloli'i, Hawaii. He learned Hawaiian Pidgin English and the Hawaiian culture during his time there.

In 2006, Steven became the Director of the MDM Observatory in Sells, Arizona, USA. Working for Columbia University and later, Dartmouth College, he developed the facility to modern standards. He learned an appreciation of the native Americans and their culture from the Tohono O'odham Nation.

In 2008, Steven joined the solar power revolution that was sweeping the USA and commissioned the largest CIGS thin film solar photovoltaic installation in the world.

A year later he commissioned the largest solar photovoltaic power plant in the USA. The system rated power was quoted as 25MW with over 90,500 solar modules that were mounted to 158 single-axis tracker systems in three hundred acres of land.

In 2010 he started to research radiation and publish the leading books on the subject. Some of the discoveries that Steven made during his independent research are:

- Found the links between solar radiation and human health issues.
- Found the links between artificial radiation and human health issues.
- "Archimedes Death Ray" effect in architecture.
- Unnaturally high levels of solar radiation in modern human society.
- Tree canopy light interference.

- Light modification by plants.
- Radiation suppression by nature.
- Structure light interference.
- The causes of power-line illness and disease.
- Atmospheric energy interference for solar radiation.
- Developed the solar photovoltaic power equations.
- Found the sources of solar photovoltaic power system overloading.

He went on to develop the solar photovoltaic team for a large international company.

Steven Magee is now one of the leading radiation and human health experts in the world and is providing consulting services to the industry. He is trained in human health, biomedical systems, astrophysics, optics and engineering.

Author Contact

Steven Magee,

3618 S. Desert Lantern Road,

Tucson,

AZ 85735,

USA

I hope that you found the book informative and please let me know about any questions or comments about the book.

I am a consultant on light and please feel free to contact me for any help or assistance.

You may find my other books useful:

Solar Photovoltaic

- Solar Photovoltaics for Consumers, Utilities and Investors
- Solar Photovoltaic Training for Residential, Commercial and Utility Systems
- Solar Photovoltaic Design for Residential, Commercial and Utility Systems

- Solar Photovoltaic Operation and Maintenance for Residential, Commercial and Utility Systems
- Solar Photovoltaic DC Calculations for Residential, Commercial and Utility Systems
- Solar Photovoltaic Resource for Residential, Commercial and Utility Systems

Solar

- Solar Irradiance and Insolation for Power Systems
- Solar Site Selection for Power Systems

Architecture

- Solar Reflections for Architects, Engineers and Human Health

Human Health

- Solar Radiation – A Cause of Illness and Cancer?
- Solar Radiation, Global Warming and Human Disease
- Toxic Light

Religion

- Solar Radiation, the Book of Revelations and the Era of Light – Part 1

You can search "Steven Magee Books" for the very latest publications.

Made in the USA
San Bernardino, CA
22 February 2013